全国高等医药院校药学类实验教材

中药炮制学实验

（第二版）

主　编　王延年

编　者　马跃平　江玲玲

中国健康传媒集团

中国医药科技出版社

内 容 提 要

本书为"全国高等医药院校药学类实验教材"之一。全书分为两章，分别为基本知识和中药炮制实验，其中中药炮制实验部分由 18 个实验组成，实验内容包括了传统实验和现代实验。为适应教育国际化的要求，增加了英文对照内容，以便于学生在阅读英文文献、撰写英文论文时参考。

本书可供高等医药院校中药学专业、中药制药专业及中药资源与开发专业使用，也可作为医药行业相关人员培训用书。

图书在版编目（CIP）数据

中药炮制学实验/王延年主编．—2 版．—北京：中国医药科技出版社，2019.10

全国高等医药院校药学类实验教材

ISBN 978 - 7 - 5214 - 1376 - 2

Ⅰ．①中…　Ⅱ．①王…　Ⅲ．①中药炮制学 - 实验 - 医学院校 - 教材　Ⅳ．①R283 - 33

中国版本图书馆 CIP 数据核字（2019）第 211821 号

美术编辑　陈君杞

版式设计　郭小平

出版　**中国健康传媒集团** | 中国医药科技出版社

地址　北京市海淀区文慧园北路甲 22 号

邮编　100082

电话　发行：010 - 62227427　邮购：010 - 62236938

网址　www. cmstp. com

规格　787 × 1092mm ¹⁄₁₆

印张　7

字数　129 千字

初版　2014 年 8 月第 1 版

版次　2019 年 10 月第 2 版

印次　2019 年 10 月第 1 次印刷

印刷　北京市密东印刷有限公司

经销　全国各地新华书店

书号　ISBN 978 - 7 - 5214 - 1376 - 2

定价　**20. 00 元**

获取新书信息、投稿、为图书纠错，请扫码联系我们。

前 言

中药炮制学是研究中药炮制理论、工艺、规格标准、历史沿革及其发展方向的综合性的应用学科，是中药学专业课程的重要组成部分。中药炮制实验是中药炮制学教学过程中的重要环节，其目的在于验证、巩固课堂讲授的内容，通过典型药物的炮制与理化检测，掌握中药炮制技术、工艺及现代中药炮制研究方法，培养学生科学的工作方法和独立思考、比较分析、综合运用知识解决问题的能力。

本实验指导是第二版修订教材，是在第一版的基础上，对不合理的内容框架进行适当调整，对不科学的内容进行纠正修改，并替换已过时的实验。根据教学大纲的要求，本书实验内容包括传统实验与现代实验部分。全书共分两章。第一章为基本知识，主要介绍了中药炮制实验的基本方法、基本要求及注意事项等。第二章为实验内容，共 18 个实验，包括传统炮制方法实验如清炒法、加固体辅料炒法、炙法、煅法、复制法、煨法、水飞法、制霜法、发酵、发芽法；综合性实验如山楂不同炮制品总有机酸、总黄酮含量的测定、槐米的炮制及其各炮制品中鞣质的含量测定、生枳壳与麸炒枳壳中总挥发油的含量及薄层鉴别比较、延胡索的炮制及炮制前后药理作用比较、炮制对黄连化学成分的影响、利用薄层色谱法检测不同软化方法对黄芩中黄芩苷的影响、煮法及乌头煮制前后乌头碱毒性的变化、巴豆制霜前后巴豆油的含量测定、发酵炮制对淡豆豉中异黄酮的影响以及综合设计实验等。最后附录内容，按炮制方法分类，以汉英对照的方式列出了中药炮制实验中的常用术语。

本书具有较强的系统性、针对性、实用性、创新性等特点，在继承中药传统炮制原则和方法的基础上，努力创新，重视现代炮制理论及方法研究的新成果、新方法，在内容和形式上都有新的突破。

本书的编写，得到沈阳药科大学教务处的大力支持，得到沈阳药科大学中药炮制学专业同学的帮助，在此致以衷心的感谢！

双语教学已成为我国当前高等医药院校教育改革的一个亮点。中药炮制学是一门既传统而又新兴的学科，开展双语教学，既是时代发展的要求，也是为了培养国际化中医药人才的需要。由于编者水平有限，书中存在一定的疏漏、不足之处，恳请读者批评指正。

编者

2019 年 8 月

目 录

第一章 基本知识

Chapter 1　Elementary Knowledge

第一节　中药炮制实验的基本方法

中药炮制是中华民族宝贵的文化财富。在几千年的中药产生、发展史上，我国劳动人民不仅积累了丰富的炮制方法和技术，而且也形成了一套传统的加工设备。中药炮制是中药学的重要组成部分，是通过加热或辅料的作用改变药性的制药技术。药物经过炮制，可以降低或消除毒副作用，保证用药安全，改变药性，利于贮存等。

中药炮制方法主要有清炒法、加固体辅料炒法、炙法、煅法、复制法、煨法、水飞法、制霜法、发酵法、发芽法及其他方法。下面列出中药炮制实验中一些常用的炮制方法。

1. 净选加工　净选加工是中药炮制第一道工序，是中药材切制成饮片或制剂前的基础工作，也是保证饮片质量的关键一环。包括清除杂质、水洗等操作。

清除杂质指清除泥浆及杂质和非药物的部分，使药物洁净或便于进一步加工处理。水洗是将药物通过水洗或漂去杂质的常用方法。

2. 饮片切制　饮片切制是根据不同的要求，将药材切制成不同规格的饮片，其目的是便于有效成分煎出、利于进一步炮炙、利于调配和贮存等。

饮片切制前，一般需要进行药材软化。药材软化的目的主要是使药材吸收一定量的水分，使药物质地由硬变软，便于切制。药材软化通常用浸泡、喷雾、洗、漂等方法。漂法是将中药材用多量水，多次漂洗的方法。古代常用长流水漂。操作时，将药材放入大量的清水中，每日频繁换水，漂去有毒成分降低其毒性，除去盐分及腥臭异味，使药物纯净。

3. 炒法　药物经净制或切制后，加辅料或不加辅料，置预热容器内，用适当火力连续加热，并不断翻动或转动，炒至一定程度标准的炮制方法，称为炒法。药物经过炒制，会改变其药性，改变或消除不良气味，增强疗效，有些药物炒后产生焦香气味，可增强健脾开胃消食的作用。药物经炒制后，失去部分水分，质地变酥脆，有利于粉碎而便于制剂，利于煎出有效成分。根据医疗用药要求，结合药物性质与炒制时加辅料与否，炒法可分为清炒法和加固体辅料炒法。

清炒法：将净制或切制后的饮片，不加辅料，置预热炒制容器内，加热翻动或转动炒至一定程度要求的方法，称为清炒法。根据炒制药物时火力及程度标准要求不同，可分为炒黄、炒焦和炒炭。炒黄的主要目的是增强疗效，降低毒性或副作用，缓和药物性能，保存药效，利于制剂和贮存。炒焦的目的主要是增强药物消食健脾止泻的功能、缓和药物的性能，减少药物的刺激性，产生焦香气味。炒炭是将净选或切制后的药物，用武火或中火炒至药物表面焦黑色或焦褐色，内部呈棕褐色或棕黄色。炒炭时只能使药物部分炭化，更不能灰化。经炒炭炮制后可使药物保存、增强或产生止血作用。

加辅料炒法：净制或切制后的饮片与固体辅料共同加热拌炒的方法，称为加辅料炒法。根据固体辅料的种类不同，可以分为麸炒、米炒、土炒、砂炒、蛤粉炒和滑石粉炒等。

4. 炙法 将净选或切制后的药物，加入一定量的液体辅料拌炒，使辅料逐渐渗入药物组织内部的炮制方法称为炙法。

药物吸入液体辅料经加工炒制后在性味、功效、作用趋向、归经和理化性质方面均能发生某些变化，起到降低毒性，抑制偏性，增强疗效，矫臭矫味，使有效成分易于溶出等作用，从而达到最大限度地发挥疗效。炙法根据所用辅料不同，可分为酒炙、醋炙、盐炙、蜜炙、姜炙、油炙等方法。

由于使用辅料是不同的，其影响也是不同的。例如，酒炙可以促进血液循环，减少一些药物的副作用；醋炙更能发挥显著影响舒缓肝脏和缓解疼痛，减少毒性作用；盐炙将加强对补肾脏的影响、滋养阴和降低火等；蜜炙润肺，有更好地影响和缓解咳嗽、补肾益胃和脾脏，或者可以适度的药品属性和降低毒性；姜炙可以更明显地影响减轻冷、呕吐和降低毒性。

5. 煅法 将药物直接或间接放入无烟炉火中或置适当的耐火容器内煅烧的方法，称为煅法。目的使其质地疏松，利于粉碎和有效成分的溶出，减少或消除副作用，提高疗效或产生新的功效。一些天然草药、矿物药或贝壳可直接燃烧，直到它们彻底变红，然后迅速放入醋、净水或药物提取液中，被称为淬。

6. 蒸法、煮法、焯法

（1）蒸法 是利用水蒸气加热药物的方法，如黄芩的蒸制。现代研究表明，黄芩遇冷水变绿，就是由于黄芩中所含的酶在一定温度和湿度下，可酶解黄芩中所含的黄芩苷，继而氧化而变绿。黄芩苷的水解又与酶的活性有关，以冷水浸，酶的活性最大。而蒸法可破坏酶，使其活性消失，有利于黄芩苷的保存。

（2）煮法 是利用清水或药汁在沸腾温度条件下加热药物，一般需煮至药透汤尽，其主要目的都是为了降低毒性或副作用。例如，煮法可以降低乌头等药物的毒副作用，并可增强药效，改变药性。乌头的毒性成分主要为双酯型生物碱，煮制后双酯型生物碱被水解形成单酯型生物碱及非酯型生物碱，其毒性分别为双酯型乌头碱的 $1/500 \sim 1/200$ 及 $1/4000 \sim 1/2000$，从而降低毒性。

（3）焯法 是在沸水中短时间（$5 \sim 10$ 分钟）浸煮的方法。焯法可以利于保存药物有效成分，去除非药用部位，或分离不同药用部位。例如，苦杏仁止咳平喘的有效成分是苦杏仁苷，易被共存的苦杏仁酶和野樱酶水解。通过焯制可以杀酶保苷，有利于保存药效，而且焯制后便于去除种皮。

7. 发酵与发芽 发酵法经净制或处理后的药物，在一定的温度和湿度条件下，由于霉菌和酶的催化分解作用，使药物发泡、生衣的方法。发芽法将净选后的新鲜成熟的果实或种子，在一定的温度或湿度条件下，促使萌发幼芽的方法。

8. 其他制法　还有一些其他特殊处理方法炮制中药，如制霜法、水飞、煨法等。

总体上，中药炮制的目的有以下几个方面：降低或消除毒副作用，保证用药安全，如草乌、川乌、附子、半夏、天南星等，通过炮制，可以降低这些中药的毒性。僵蚕具有化痰散结之功，但容易引起呕吐，经麸炒炮制后可以减少这些副作用。

中药炮制提高治疗效果。例如，紫菀、枇杷叶蜂蜜炙能促进润肺来缓解咳嗽，当归、川芎经酒炮制能促进血液循环，延胡索用醋炙可以加强镇痛的作用。

中药炮制可以改变中药的药性，使他们适合的治疗需求。例如，生首乌具有泻下润燥等功效，炮制后更擅于补益肝肾作用。

中药炮制还可以清除杂质、非药用部分和不良气味，使中药材更加纯净，方便患者服用。

大多数植物草药后切成段或块，其有效成分容易溶解在水中，或利于制剂。中药中大多数矿物和贝壳，煅烧或淬火用醋后，很容易被粉碎。一些中药经过炮制和干燥，可以保持很长一段时间，避免发霉、腐烂。

Section 1　Basic Experimental Methods of Traditional Chinese Medicine Processing

Processing is an important cultural treasure of China. In the past several thousand years, Chinese have not only accumulated abundant methods and technologies for processing, but also formed a set of traditional processing instruments.

Processing of traditional Chinese medicine (TCM) is one of the important part of traditional Chinese medicine. It is the technique of altering the properties of crude medicines by processing using heat and combination with various materials in a kind of alchemical approach to preparation. Processing of TCM, can promote therapeutic effects, reduce their toxicity, change their nature and effects and are easily stored.

TCM processing methods may involve such means as stir – frying drugs without adjuvant, stir – frying drugs with solid adjuvant, stir – frying with liquid adjuvant, calcined method, steaming, boiling, scalding, repeatedly processing, roasting, purification and the method of refining powder with water, and other methods.

There are several common processing methods which often be used in the processing experiment are listed briefly as following.

1. Processing method of purifying

Processing method of purifying is the first step of TCM processing. It is key link to ensure the quality of TCM slices, is also the basis work of Chinese herbal medicine before the drugs are cut into slices or preparations. In general, processing method of purifying include discarding impurity or washing method. Discarding impurity refer to take away the impurity, the mud and non – pharmaceutical parts, thus making the herbs clean and pure. Washing is a kind of method of treating crude drug materials for the purposes of cleaning. Impurity and mud on the surface of the crude drug materials should be cleaned with water.

2. Processing method of cutting

According to different requirements, cut crude drug materials into pieces, parts or tiny bit, etc. , for convenience in decocting or further preparing, drying, and storing, etc. .

The crude drug materials usually need to be softened before it was cut. Softening is a kind of method of treating crude drug materials in order to attain the purposes of making them easy to cut. This method often include sprinkling, washing, soaking – with – sealing with clean water so as to make them soften or easy to cut.

Rinsing is a method for removing the salty elements, poisonous substances, offensive smell from the crude drugs by laying them a certain time in a large container with water. During the Rinsing, water must be changed frequently. The method of Rinsing is a kind of method of treating crude drug materials for the purposes of cleaning, softening, regulating medicinal properties or making them easy to cut, or reducing their toxicity, or making drugs pure, etc. .

3. Stir – frying (Processing with fire)

By stir – frying, the properties and effects of crude drugs can be properly changed, their irritant properties and side – effects can be reduced and their side – nature of coldness or dryness may be moderated. Stir – frying crude drug materials have the actions of checking offensive odor and tastes and invigorating the spleen, and they are easy to be pounded into pieces or powder and stored, and their effective components may be dissolved or extracted easily . Stir – frying drugs may be divided into two methods, stir – frying without adjuvants and stir – frying with solid adjuvants.

Stir – frying without adjuvants is the procedure of stir – baking without adjuvants. According to the degrees required, the method of stir – frying without adjuvants can be divided into three kinds, stir – frying crude drug materials until they become yellowish; stir – frying crude drug materials until they become burnt – colorand stir – frying crude drug materials until they become carbonized.

By stir – frying crude drug materials into yellowish, it means that they are stir – frying into yellow surface or till they bulge while there is no change in their interior. Stir – frying crude drug materials into yellowish can reduce the coldness and side – effect. By stir – frying crude drug materials into burnt – color, it means that they are toasted into burnt – yellow or burnt – brown surface and yellow interior with burnt odor. Stir – frying drugs into burnt – color can promote the action of invigorating the spleen and digestion. By stir – frying drugs into carbonized, it means that their surface becomes burnt black and the interior is burnt yellow while their medicinal properties or form still exist. After stir – frying, their function of arresting hemorrhage can be reinforced.

Stir – frying with solid adjuvants is the procedure of stir – frying with certain amount of solid adjuvants until the degrees required. The commonly – used adjuvants are wheat bran, rice, mud, sand, pulverized – clamshell, etc..

4. Stir – frying with liquid adjuvants

The commonly – used liquid adjuvants include wine, vinegar, salt solution, honey, ginger juice and oil, etc.. The purpose of this method is to increase their therapeutic actions, to correct their pharmaceutical properties, or reduce their side – effects through gradual increase of permeation of the liquid adjuvants into the medicinal materials during processing.

The different liquid adjuvants which used in process will lead to different effects on crude drug materials. For example, wine – stir – frying drugs can promote the blood circulation and reduce the side – effects of some pharmaceutical herbs; vinegar – stir – frying drugs can exert more remarkable effects on soothing the liver and relieving pain and reducing the toxic effects; salt solution – stir – frying drugs will strengthen the effects on tonifying the kidney, nourishing yin and lowering the fire; honey – stir – frying traditional Chinese medicinal have better effects on moistening the lung and relieving cough, invigorating the stomach and spleen, or can moderate the pharmaceutical properties and reduce the toxic effects; ginger juice – stir – frying drugs can get more obvious effects on relieving cold, vomiting and reducing the toxic effects, etc..

The methods of stir – frying with liquid adjuvants are respectively known as stir – frying with wine, vinegar, salt solution, honey and ginger juice.

5. Calcining

It is a method of treating crude drug materials by direct or indirect burning with medium heating fire or strong fire. The purposes of calcining is to make them pure, clean, crispy, easy to be powdered and their effective components is apt to extracted. Calcining method can change natures of crude drug materials to increase therapeutic effects.

Some crude drug materials of hard minerals or shells may be burned directly till they are thoroughly reddish, then they are quickly put into clean water(this method is called water – tempering) or vinegar(this method is called vinegar – tempering), which is called tempering.

6. Steaming, Boiling, Scalding(Processing with both fire and water)

Steaming is a method of processing crude drug materials by putting them in a steaming pot or other container to heat them with steam. For example, steaming of Radix Scutellariae can reserve most baicalin because steaming processing can destroy the enzyme to protect the baicalin.

Boiling is a method of treating the crude drug materials by heating them in clean water or other liquid adjuvants at boiling temperature. The main purpose is to detoxify. For example, The toxic constituent of aconite root is alkaloid which posses double ester bonds, and can be hydrolyzed to single ester bond alkaloid or diester type alkaloid by boiling, which toxicity is $1/500 \sim 1/200$ or $1/4000 \sim 1/2000$ of that double ester bonds type, respectively.

Scalding is a method of treating the crude drug materials by putting them into boiling water, and stirring them for a short time ($5 \sim 10$ minutes), take them out as the seed coats are expanded and soak in cold water. Take them out and separate the seed coat and kernel by rubbing.

Scalding method is facilitate to preserve effective component, remove the non – medicinal part, or separate the different medicinal parts. For example, Bitter apricot kernel contains amygdalin, which is the active constituent for relieving cough and asthma. Amygdalin can be enzymolyse by amygdalase. Scalding can inactivate the enzyme to avoid the enzymatic hydrolysis of amygdalin and then enhance the clinical effect, and be convenient for removing the seed coat.

7. Fermentation and Germination

Fermentation means that pharmaceutical crude materials are fermented at certain temperature with a series of procedures. Germination means that crude drug materials seeds are germinated to certain highness.

8. Other processing methods

There are some other special processing methods according to different requirement of crude drug materials, such as frost – like powder, levigation, roasting, etc. .

As a whole, the purposes of processing traditional Chinese medicinal are briefly summarized as follows.

Removing or reducing the toxicity, drastic properties and side effects of some Chinese medicinal herbs. For instance, the poisonous components of medicinal herbs, such as Radix Aconiti Kusnezoffii (Caowu) , Radix Aconiti (Chuanwu) , Radix Euphorbiae Kansui (Gansui) , Rhizoma Pinelliae (Banxia) and Rhizoma Arisaematis (Tiannanxing) , will be reduced when they are processed; Bombyx Batryticatus (Jiangcan) , after taken, easily induce vomiting and if used to reducing phlegm and resolving masses, the side effects can be reduced after stir – frying with wheat bran.

Processing of traditional Chinese medicine can promote therapeutic effects. For instance, radix asteris (Ziwan) , Folium Eriobotryae (Pipaye) roasted with honey can promote nourishing the lung to relieve cough; Rhizoma Chuanxiong (Chuanxiong) and Radix Angelicae Sinensis (Danggui) stir – frying with wine can promote warming channels to promote blood circulation; Rhizoma Corydalis (Yanhusuo) prepared with vinegar can strengthen the effects of relieving pain.

Modifying the natures and actions of traditional Chinese medicinal so as to make them suitable for therapeutic requirements. For instance, Radix Polygoni (Heshouwu) in raw form has moistening – purging effect, but after processed by steaming method, it can be good at invigorating the liver and kidney.

Processing of traditional Chinese medicine can taking away the impurity, non – pharmaceutical parts and unpleasant tastes, thus making traditional Chinese medicine clean and pure, and convenient for patients to take.

Most traditional Chinese medicine will be easily decocted in water after cut into pieces or segments and their effective components will be easily dissolved out or the forms of drugs will be easily prepared. Most of shells and minerals of Chinese medicinal herbs, will be easy to be ground into powder after calcined or quenched with vinegar. Some medicinal herbs are to be stir – fried and fully dried so as to be kept for a long time from being moldy or rot.

第二节 中药炮制实验基本要求及注意事项

中药炮制实验室是中药炮制课程的一个重要组成部分。用于加深对中药炮制知识的理解；全面了解中药炮制工作的性质和任务，培养严肃认真、实事求是的科学态度和工作作风。

实验课程要求学生熟练掌握各种炮制方法和操作技术，培养独立开展中药炮制工作的能力。正确掌握实验教材中各类代表性药物的炮制方法。为确保实验教学质量，每个实验者应认真做到以下几点：

（1）实验前做好预习，明确实验的目的和要求，熟悉原理和操作要点，估计实验中可能发生的问题及处理方法，有准备地接受教师的提问。

（2）为防止试剂、药品污染，取用时应仔细观察标签，杜绝错盖瓶盖或不随手加盖的现象发生。当不慎发生试剂污染时，应及时报告任课教师。公用试剂、药品应在指定位置取用。此外，取出的试剂、药品不能再倒回原瓶。

（3）及时做好完整而确切的原始记录。要用钢笔或圆珠笔书写，字体端正。应直接记录于实验记录本上，不允许记于纸条上或者其他本子上。

（4）爱护仪器，小心使用，破损仪器应及时报损、补发。动用精密仪器，须经教师同意，用后登记签名。

（5）严格按照实验规程操作，细心观察实验现象。认真总结实验数据，按指定格式填写实验报告，并按规定时间上交。

（6）爱护公物，节约水电、药品和试剂。可回收利用的废溶剂应回收至指定的容器中，不可随意弃去。腐蚀性残液应倒入废液缸中，切勿倒进水槽。

（7）实验时确保安全，时刻注意防火、防爆。发现可能的事故及时报告，不懂时不要擅自动手处理。

（8）实验完毕应认真清理实验台，仪器洗净后放回原处，擦净台面，经指导教师同意后，方可离开。值日生还应负责整理公用试剂台、打扫地面卫生、清除垃圾及废液缸中的废物，并检查水、电、门窗等安全事宜。

Section 2　Basic Requirements and Announcements in Experiment of Traditional Chinese Medicine Processing

Processing of traditional Chinese medicine experimental course is an important part of Processing of Chinese herbal medicinals subject. Its purpose is to deepen the comprehension of Processing of traditional Chinese herbal medicinals knowledge, to have full understanding of the property and task of the work, and to develop serious, practical and realistic scientific attitude and work style.

The experimental course claim students to expertly grasp various analytical methods and operational technique. It will also train students to have the ability to carry out the processing of traditional Chinese herbal medicinals work indepengdently, and to master the processing method of each kind of representative medicine in the experimental book accurately. To sure the quality of experimental teaching, every experimenter should observe the terms seriously as follows:

(1) Preview the experiment content seriously before carrying out an experiment. Make good understanding of the experimental purpose and demands, be familiar with the principle, experimental procedures. Full consideration should be given to the precaution of accident and to the settlement of the accident happened in any case, prepare to answer the questions which teacher should ask.

(2) To prevent reagents and drugs pollution, carefully observe the label of them before using. Eradicate the occurrence of covering a wrong bottle capping or without cover after use reagents. While the immodesty reagents pollution occurrence, be sure to report to teachers in time. The public reagents, drugs should be used at appointed place. In addition, reagent and drugs taken out must not be poured back to original bottle.

(3) Record original experiment date directly in experimental record notebook in time completely and accurately. Write with fountain pen or ball – pen. Forbid to record on note paper of other books.

(4) Take good care of equipment, use carefully, in case the instruments damaged, register and report to replacing in time. It must be obtained by teacher, and be sure to register the signature after usage.

(5) Perform the experiment strictly according to the experimental procedures, observe experiment phenomena carefully. Summary experimental result seriously. Fill in the experiment report according to appoint format, hand in report on schedule.

(6) Take good care of public property, economize the electricity, water, drugs and reagents. Waste solvent which can be recovered should be poured into the appointed container. It must not be leaved arbitrarily. Causticity aqua should be poured into waste liquor cistern, absolutely do not pour into the sink.

(7) Guarantee the safety during experiment. Pay attention to prevent from fire and explosion all the time. Any indication of trouble should be reported in time. Do not do any disposal if you can not deal with correctly.

(8) After the experiment, clean up the experiment bench, all the instruments used should be cleaned and put in order. With all above been done and the tutor's permission students can leave the laboratory. Students on duty should clean the public agent bench, floor, rubbish and the dirty in waste liquor cistern. Check the water, electricity, door and windows finally.

第二章　中药炮制实验

Chapter 2　Experiment for Processing of Traditional Chinese Medicine

实验一　清炒法

【实验目的】

1. 掌握清炒法的目的和意义。

2. 掌握炒黄、炒焦、炒炭的基本操作方法及饮片质量要求。

3. 掌握炒黄、炒焦、炒炭 3 种炒法的不同火力、火候，炒后药性的变化及炒炭"存性"的含义。

【实验原理】

炒法分为清炒和加辅料炒两种。根据炒法所用的的火力、火候不同，清炒法又分为炒黄、炒焦和炒炭。炒黄多用"文火"，炒焦多用"中火"，炒炭多用"武火"。

炒制的目的是为了改变药性，提高疗效，降低毒性和减少副作用，矫味、矫臭及便于制剂等。

【实验器材】

铁锅、炉子、铁铲、瓷盆、筛子、温度计、竹匾、天平等。

【实验内容】

1. **炒黄（炒爆）**　　目的：增强疗效，缓和药性，降低毒性，并破坏某些药物中的酶，以保存苷类成分（杀酶保苷）。

（1）莱菔子　取净莱菔子，用文火炒至鼓起，有爆裂声，并有香气逸出时，取出放凉。用时捣碎。

成品性状：本品呈类圆形或椭圆形而稍扁，表面黄棕色或红棕色或灰褐色，味辛苦，炒后鼓起，色泽加深，具油香气。

炮制作用：生品涌吐风痰；制品降气化痰，消食导滞（生升熟降）。

（2）王不留行（炒爆）　　先将锅烧热，投入王不留行，中火不断翻炒至大部分（80%）爆成白花，迅速取出放凉。

成品性状：本品呈圆球形，黑色或黑棕色，略有光泽，味微甘，炒后鼓起，80%以上爆裂成白色爆花，体轻质脆。

炮制作用：生品消痈肿；炮制后易于煎出有效成分，且走散力增强。

注意事项：锅要预热，中火炒制，可先投少量试锅，不断翻炒，出锅迅速，要求：80%以上爆成白花。（王不留行名字来源：性善走而不守，虽有王命不能留其行。）

（3）决明子　取净决明子，置炒制容器内，用文火加热，炒至微有爆裂声，并有香气逸出，取出放凉，用时捣碎。

成品性状：炒决明子种皮破裂，颜色加深，偶有焦斑，质稍脆，微有香气。

炮制作用：生品长于清肝热，润肠燥；炒制后寒泻之性缓和，有平肝养肾的功效。

（4）酸枣仁　取净酸枣仁，称重，置热锅内，用文火炒至鼓起微有爆裂声，颜色微变深，并嗅到药香气时，出锅放凉。用时捣碎。

成品性状：本品呈紫红色，鼓起，有裂纹，无焦斑，手捻种皮易脱落。具香气。

2. **炒焦**　目的：增强疗效，减小药物刺激性。

（1）山楂　取净山楂，用中火加热，炒至外表焦褐色，内部焦黄色，取出放凉。

成品性状：本品炒焦后，表面呈焦褐色，内部焦黄色，酸味略减，微香。

炮制作用：生品长于活血化瘀；炒焦后可缓和对胃的刺激性，长于消食化积。

（2）麦芽　取净麦芽，称重，置热锅内，先用文火后用中火加热，不断翻动，炒至表面焦褐色，喷淋少许清水，炒干取出，放凉。筛去碎屑。

成品性状：本品呈焦褐色，膨胀，少部分爆花。

炮制作用：炒焦后增强助消化作用。

（3）槟榔　取净槟榔片，称重，分档，置热锅内，用文火加热，不断翻炒至焦黄色，有焦斑，取出放凉。筛去碎屑。

成品性状：本品大部分为完整片状，表面焦黄色，具焦斑。有香气。

炮制作用：炒焦后降低副作用。

3. **炒炭**　目的：使药物增强或产生止血作用（炒炭要求"存性"）。

（1）山楂　取净山楂，用武火加热，炒至表面焦黑色，内部焦褐色，取出放凉。

成品性状：本品炒炭后，表面呈焦黑色，内部焦褐色，味涩。

炮制作用：生品长于活血化瘀；炒炭后止血止泻。

（2）地榆　取净地榆片，武火炒至外表焦褐色，内部棕褐色，取出放凉。

成品性状：本品炒炭后呈黑褐色，味涩。

炮制作用：生品以凉血解毒力胜；炒炭后长于收敛止血。

（3）槐米　取净槐米，称重，置热锅内，用中火加热不断翻炒至黑褐色，发现火星，可喷淋适量清水熄灭，炒干，取出放凉。

成品性状：本品表面呈焦黑色，保留原药外形，存性。

【**实验记录**】

（1）记录炒黄、炒焦和炒炭中各种药物形态、颜色、气味的变化。

（2）记录实验中出现的问题并说明原因。

【**注意事项**】

（1）药物炒制前应按照大小分档，根据不同炒法及其要求控制火候、时间，注意药材外观的变化。如：酸枣仁炒黄时火力不宜过强，且炒的时间也不宜过久，否则油枯失效。王不留行翻炒不宜过快，否则影响其爆花率及爆花程度。

（2）炒制操作过程中，要勤翻动，使药物受热均匀，避免生熟不均的现象。

（3）炒黄防止焦化，炒焦防止炭化，炒炭防止灰化。

（4）炒炭要注意防火，如炒制过程中出现火星，应喷洒适量清水，熄灭火星，并炒干后方可出锅。

【思考题】

（1）炒黄、炒焦、炒炭的操作要点是什么，有哪些注意事项？

（2）炒炭多用武火，为何槐米炒炭要用"中火"？试以炒黄为例，说明在炒制过程中，如何掌握火候。

（3）解释炒炭"存性"的含义及意义。

Experiment 1　Stir – frying Drugs without Adjuvant

Purpose

1. To understand the processing purpose of stir – frying drugs without adjuvant.

2. To master the processing method of stir – frying drugs without adjuvant, including stir – frying drug to yellow, stir – frying drug to brown and stir – frying drug to charcoal.

3. To master the heating strength and degree of stir – frying drug to yellow, stir – frying drug to brown and stir – frying drug to charcoal, to understand the meaning of preserving the nature of the drug after stir – frying drug to charcoal.

Principle

The processing methods of stir – frying drugs in a caldron include stir – frying drugs without adjuvant and stir – frying with adjuvant. According to different firing strength and degree of heating, the processing method of stir – frying drugs without adjuvant include stir – frying drug to yellow, stir – frying drug to brown and stir – frying drug to charcoal. Usually, stir – frying drug to yellow needs mild heating fire, stir – frying drug to brown needs medium heating, and stir – frying drug to charcoal needs strong heating fire.

The purposes of stir – frying drugs can be briefly summarized as follows, removing or reducing the toxicity, promoting therapeutic effects, taking away the impurity, non – pharmaceutical parts and unpleasant tastes, drastic properties and side – effects of some Chinese medicinal herbs.

Instruments

Pot, stove, shovel, ceramic bowl, sieve, thermometer, split – bamboo basket, balance etc. .

Experimental Contents

1. Stir – frying drug to yellow

（1）Raphani Semen（Laifuzi）

Processing method：Put the clean Semen Raphani in hot pot, heat with mild heating fire, stir – frying continuously until the drugs inflated, produce crack, and have aromatic. Chill before serving. Break them into pieces before using.

Characteristics of finished products：The stir – fried drugs have darker color, expand slightly, have fragrance, have pungent and bitter taste.

Effect of processing: The crude drug mainly has the function of promoting spit wind – phlegm. The stir – fried drug mainly has the function of depressing qi and reducing phlegm, helping to digest and guiding lag. (The crude drugs pertain to ascending while cooked drugs pertain to descending.)

(2) Vaccariae Semen(Wangbuliuxing)

Processing method: Put the clean Semen Vaccariae in hot pot, heat with medium heating fire, stir continuously until most of the drugs burst into white flowers, remove from the pot quickly. Chill before serving.

Characteristics of finished products: More than 80% of the stir – fried drugs burst into white flowers, crisp.

Effect of processing: The crude drug mainly has the function of eliminating carbuncle swollen. The active ingredient is apt to extract after the drugs become puffed.

Matters needing attention: Preheat the pot before the drugs were put in, heat with medium heating fire.

(3) Cassiae Semen(Juemingzi)

Processing method: Put the clean Semen Cassiae in hot pot, heat with mild heating fire, stir continuously until the drugs produce crack, and have aromatic. Chill before serving. Break them into pieces before using.

Characteristics of finished products: The stir – fried drugs have darker color, expand slightly, have focal spot occasionally, have fragrance.

Effect of processing: The crude drug is good at eliminating liver heat, lubricating the intestines. The character of cold diarrhea is alleviated, has the function of calming the liver and nourishing the kidney after it was sair – fried.

(4) Ziziphi Spinosae Semen(Suanzaoren)

Processing method: Put the clean Semen Ziziphi spinosae in hot pot, heat with mild heating fire, stir continuously until the drugs inflated, color slightly darken, produce crack, and have aromatic. Chill before serving. Break them into pieces before using.

Characteristics of finished products: The stir – fried drugs have amaranth color, fragrance, expand slightly, without focal spot.

Effect of processing: The active ingredient is apt to extract after the drugs stir – fried. It benefit for promoting therapeutic effects.

2. Stir – frying drug to brown

(1) Crataegi Fructus(Shanzha)

Processing method: Put the clean Crataegi Fructus slices in hot pot, heat with medium heating fire, stir continuously until the surface of drugs becomes a focal brown, and interior of drugs becomes focal yellow.

Characteristics of finished products: The surface of finished product is focal brown, and interior of finished product is focal yellow. Sour taste slightly reduced. Have fragrant slightly.

Effect of processing: The crude drug of Crataegi Fructus is good at promoting blood circulation to remove blood stasis. After processed, it will benefit for easing irritating to the stomach, good at helping digestion.

(2) Hordei Fructus Germinatus (Maiya)

Processing method (Stir – frying drug to brown): Put the clean Hordei Fructus Germinatus in hot pot, heat with medium heating fire, stir continuously until the surface of drugs becomes ustulate, spray a little water, roast dehydration, remove from the pot quickly. Chill before serving.

Characteristics of finished products: The surface of finished product is dark yellow or focal brown, expand, small part of the drugs burst into flowers, having fragrant slightly.

Effect of processing: The crude drug of Fructus Hordei Germinatus is good at promoting digestion. After stir – frying drug to brown, it is much stronger in the effects of promoting digestion.

(3) Areca Semen (Binglang)

Processing method: Put the clean Areca Semen slices in hot pot, heat with medium heating fire, stir continuously until the surface of drugs becomes focal yellow, remove from the pot quickly. Chill before serving. Screen to clastic.

Characteristics of finished products: The surface of finished product is dark yellow, having focal spot, fragrant slightly.

Effect of processing: Reduce the side – effects.

3. Stir – frying drug to charcoal

(1) Charred Crataegi Fructus (Shanzha)

Processing method: Put the clean Crataegi Fructus slices in hot pot, heat with strong fire, stir continuously until the surface of drugs becomes charred and black, and interior of drugs becomes focal brown.

Characteristics of finished products: The surface of finished product is charred and black, and interior of finished product is focal brown. The taste is puckery.

Effect of processing: The crude drug is good at promoting blood circulation to remove blood stasis. After processed, it good at hemostasis and cure diarrhea.

(2) Sanguisorbae Radix (Diyu)

Processing method: Put the clean Sanguisorbae Radix in hot pot, heat with strong fire, stir continuously until the surface of drugs becomes charred and black, and interior of drugs becomes focal brown.

Characteristics of finished products: The surface of finished product is charred and black, and interior of finished product is focal brown. The taste is puckery.

Effect of processing: The crude drug is good at cooling blood to relieve internal heat or fever. After processed, it good at astringency and hemostasis.

（3）Sophorae Flos（Huaimi）

Processing method：Put the clean Sophorae Flos in hot pot，heat with medium heating fire，stir continuously until the drugs becomes focal brown.

Characteristics of finished products：The surface of finished product is focal brown. Keep the shape of crude drug. Keep properties of the drug.

Effect of processing：Strengthen the hemostatic effect.

Experimental records

（1）Record the changes ofform，color and odour during the processing of stir－frying drug to yellow，stir－frying drug to brown and stir－frying drug to charcoal.

（2）Make a record of the problems appeard during the experiment and explain the causes of the problems.

Matters needing attention

（1）Separate the crude drugs by size before stir－frying，avoid uneven heating. During the processing，stir－fry the drug at appropriate temperature.

（2）During the process，it is necessary tostir frequently in order that the drugs is heated evenly，avoid uneven heated.

（3）Prevent scorching in the process of stir－frying drug to yellow；Prevent carbonization in the process of stir－frying drug to brown；Prevent ashing in the process of stir－frying drug to charcoal.

（4）Pay attention to fire protection in the process of stir－frying drug to charcoal. If flake is found，please spray some water to extinguish flake，stir－frying to dry before remove it from the pot.

Reflection Questions

（1）What are the operating points of stir－frying drug to yellow，stir－frying drug to brown and stir－frying drug to charcoal?

（2）Usually，stir－frying drug to charcoal needs strong heating fire，but stir－frying Flos Sophorae Immaturus to charcoal needs medium heating. How to explain it?

（3）How to understand the meaning of preserving the nature of the drug after stir－frying drug to charcoal?

实验二　山楂不同炮制品总黄酮、总有机酸含量的测定

【实验目的】

1. 掌握山楂不同炮制品山楂、炒山楂、焦山楂、山楂炭的炮制过程和操作方法。

2. 通过山楂炮制前后总有机酸和总黄酮类成分含量的变化，了解中药山楂的炮制作用和意义。

【实验原理】

中药山楂的炮制方法主要有炒黄、炒焦和炒炭等。现代研究认为，山楂中总有机

酸和黄酮类化合物具有多方面的药理作用。山楂味酸、甘、微温,具有致过敏的偏性。因此,山楂炮制的主要目的是降低酸性,缓和或减少刺激性。本实验通过山楂炮制前后总有机酸和总黄酮含量的比较,说明山楂的炮制作用。

【实验器材】

1. 仪器 9100 型分光光度计、称量瓶、分析天平、量筒、水浴锅、锥形瓶、圆底烧瓶、冷凝管、玻璃漏斗、移液管、容量瓶、吸量管、碱式滴定管、磁力搅拌器。

2. 试剂 芦丁标准品、氢氧化钠、酚酞、滤纸、乙醇、亚硝酸钠、硝酸铝。

【实验内容】

1. 山楂的炮制方法

(1) 生山楂 取原药材,除去杂质及脱落的核。

(2) 炒山楂 取净山楂,置热锅中,用文火加热,炒至色变深时,取出,放凉。

(3) 焦山楂 取净山楂,置热锅中,用中火加热,炒至表面焦褐色,内部焦黄色时,取出,放凉。

(4) 山楂炭 取净山楂,置热锅中,用武火加热,炒至表面焦黑色,内部焦褐色时,取出,放凉。

2. 总黄酮含量测定

(1) 标准曲线的制备 取干燥至恒重的芦丁对照品 1g,精密称定。加入 100 ml 量瓶中,加入适量 60% 乙醇,在水浴上加热溶解,冷却后用蒸馏水定容至刻度,摇匀,制成约 0.01mg/ml 的对照品溶液。

精密称取干燥至恒重的芦丁对照品适量,加 60% 乙醇制成 0.01mg/ml 的对照品溶液。精密吸取对照品溶液 0、1.0、2.0、3.0、4.0、5.0ml,分别置 10ml 量瓶中,加 60% 乙醇至 5ml,精密加入 10% 亚硝酸钠溶液 0.3ml,摇匀,放置 6 分钟,加 10% 硝酸铝溶液 0.3ml,放置 6 分钟,加 1mol/L 氢氧化钠溶液 4ml,用蒸馏水稀释至刻度,振摇 15 分钟。分别在 500nm 波长处测定吸收度 A,并以吸收度 A 为纵坐标,浓度 C 为横坐标绘制标准曲线。

(2) 供试品溶液的制备 分别取生山楂及其炮制品粉末 0.5g,精密称定。置圆底烧瓶中,精密加入 60% 乙醇 50ml,密塞,超声处理 30 分钟,冷却后过滤,作为供试品溶液。

(3) 总黄酮含量的测定 精密吸取三种供试品溶液 1ml,分别置试管中,加 60% 乙醇 4ml,加 10% 亚硝酸钠溶液 0.3ml,混匀,放置 6 分钟,加 10% 硝酸铝溶液 0.3ml,放置 6 分钟,加 1mol/L 氢氧化钠溶液 4ml,加蒸馏水 0.4ml,放置 15 分钟。

空白对照溶液的制备:取 60% 乙醇 5ml,加 10% 亚硝酸钠溶液 0.3ml,混匀,放置 6 分钟,加 10% 硝酸铝溶液 0.3ml,放置 6 分钟,加 1mol/L 氢氧化钠溶液 4ml,加蒸馏水 0.4ml,放置 15 分钟。

在 500nm 波长处测定吸收度,按标准曲线计算各供试品溶液中总黄酮的含量,结果填入表 2 - 1。

表 2 - 1　山楂不同炮制品中黄酮含量测定结果

样品	生山楂	炒山楂	焦山楂	山楂炭
吸光度 A				
含量				

3. 总有机酸含量测定　取山楂、炒山楂、焦山楂、山楂炭各 1g，精密称定。分别置锥形瓶中，加水 100ml，置磁力搅拌器常温搅拌 4 小时，过滤。精密吸取滤液 25ml，置锥形瓶中，加水 50ml，加酚酞指示剂 2 滴，用 0.1mol/L 氢氧化钠液滴定至终点。

每 1ml 0.1mol/L 氢氧化钠相当于 6.404mg 的枸橼酸（总有机酸含量以枸橼酸计算）。

表 2 - 2　山楂不同炮制品中总有机酸含量测定结果

样品	生山楂	炒山楂	焦山楂	山楂炭
总有机酸含量				

【实验记录】

（1）记录总黄酮含量测定、总有机酸含量测定各实验结果，分别填入表 2 - 1 和表 2 - 2。

（2）记录实验中出现的问题并说明原因。

【注意事项】

（1）按《中国药典》规定，山楂应去除脱落的核。

（2）区别山楂炒黄、炒焦和炒炭的质量标准。

（3）含量测定过程中应注意：生山楂要充分干燥；玻璃仪器应洁净干燥；9100 - 分光光度仪应预热至稳定。

【思考题】

（1）山楂为何要炮制？

（2）山楂炮制时应怎样控制炒黄、炒焦和炒炭的火力、火候？

（3）山楂中含有哪些有机酸类及黄酮类化合物？

（4）有机酸类和黄酮类化合物的含量测定方法还有哪些？

【相关资料】

山楂为蔷薇科植物山里红 *Crataegus pinnatifida* Bge. var. major N. E. Br. 或山楂 *Crataegus pinnatifida* Bge. 的干燥成熟果实，具消食健胃、行气散瘀的功能。中医药理论认为，山楂经不同方法炮制后，其功效有所改变：焦山楂善于消食，山楂炭长于收敛止血。现代研究认为，山楂中总有机酸类能促进胃中消化酶的分泌，促进消化，且含有脂肪酶，能加强脂肪酶和蛋白酶的活性，如熊果酸；黄酮类化合物对心血管疾病有显著疗效，具有扩张血管、强心、降压和降脂作用，如金丝桃苷、牡荆素等（化合物结构见图 2 - 1）。

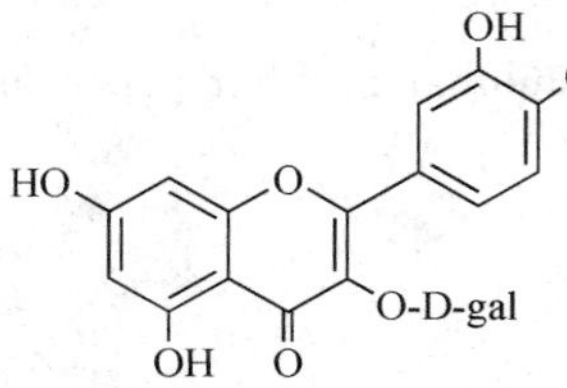

金丝桃苷

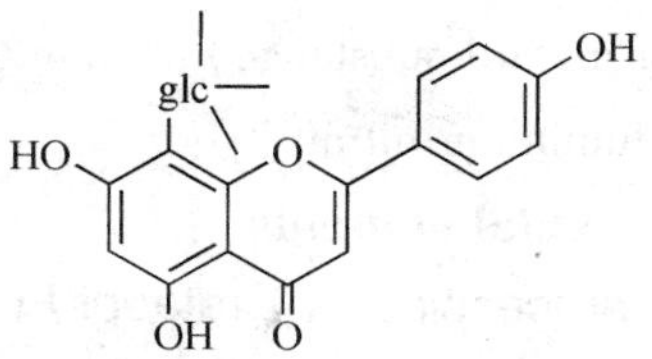

牡荆素

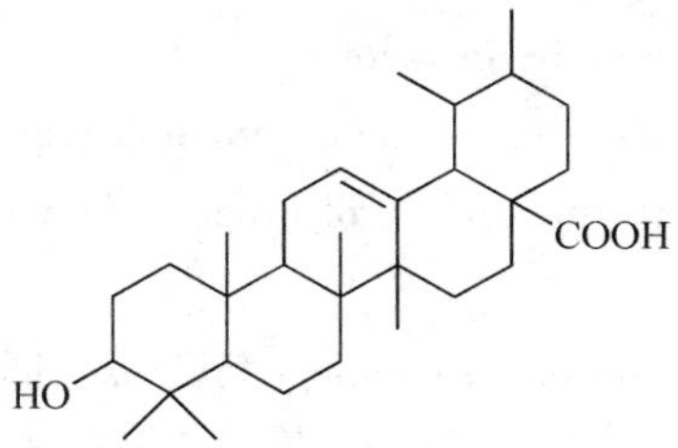

熊果酸

图 2 - 1　山楂中有机酸类、黄酮类化合物

Experiment 2　The Assay of the Total Flavone and Organic Acid in Different Processed Products of Crataegi Fructus

Purpose

1. To master the processing methods of Fructus Crataegi including stir – frying to yellow, stir – frying to brown and stir – frying to charcoal.

2. To study the assay of total flavone and organic acid and action of different processed products of Fructus Crataegi.

Principle

The usual processing methods of Crataegi Fructus including stir – fried Fructus Crataegi, charred Crataegi Fructus and charcoaled Crataegi Fructus. Modern study showed that the flavone and organic acid of charred Fructus Crataegi possess multifarious pharmacological action. The property of the crataegolic acid is sweet, slight warmth, and sourness. So the purpose of the processing about Crataegi Fructus is decreasing sourness, alleviating or reducing its irritant activity. The experiment showed that different processed products of Crataegi Fructus have important significance through the comparison of contents of the flavone and organic acid.

Instruments and chemicals

1. Instruments

9100 – specreophotomerer, weighing bottle, analytic balance, conical beaker, water – bath caudldron, dosimeter, round bottom flask, condensation tube, hyalo – runnel, transferring pipette, volumetric flask, pipette, basic burette, magnetic stirrer.

2. Chemicals

Rutin(standard substance), sodium hydroxide, phenolphthalein, filter paper, alcohol, sodium nitrite, aluminium nitrate.

Experimental contents

1. The processing of Crataegi Fructus

(1)Crataegi Fructus: Eliminate foreign matter and fallen kernels.

(2)Stir – fried Crataegi Fructus: Stir – fry the clean Fructus Crataegi as described under the method for simple stir – frying until darkens in color.

(3)Charred Crataegi Fructus: Put the clean Fructus crataegi slices in hot pot, heat with medium heating fire, stir continuously until the surface of drugs becomes a focal brown, and interior of drugs becomes focal yellow.

(4)Crataegi Fructus Charcoal: Put the clean Crataegi Fructus slices in hot pot, heat with strong fire, stir continuously until the surface of drugs becomes charred and black, and interior of drugs becomes focal brown.

2. The assay of the total flavones

(1)The preparation of standard curve: Take Rutin (drying to constant weight) 1g, weight accurately. Put into a 100ml of the volumetric flask, add proper amount of the 60% alcohol. Heated in water – bath to dissolve, diluted to the volume by distilled water after cooling and shaking. The solution concentration should be 0. 01mg/ml.

Take 0ml, 1. 0ml, 2. 0ml, 3. 0ml, 4. 0ml, 5. 0ml of the above – mentioned standard solution, accurately measured, put into 10ml volumetric flask. Add 60% of the ethyl alcohol to 5. 0ml, add 0. 3ml of sodium nitrate solution (10%) accurately, shake up. Six minutes later, add 0. 3ml of aluminium nitrate (10%) again, shake up, after laying 6 minutes, add 4ml of sodium hydroxide (1mol/L) and diluted to the volume with distilled water, shake 15 minutes. Determine the absorbance (A) at 500nm, using A as the ordinate, the abscissa is the standard solution concentration(C) as the abscissa to make the standard curve.

(2)Preparation of sample: Take about 0. 5g powder of crude drug and processed sample, weight accurately. Add to the round bottom flask, add 50ml 60% of ethyl alcohol, extract 30 minutes by supersonic in water – bath, filtrate after cooling.

(3)The assay of sample: Suck 1ml of the filtrate accurately, add to a 10ml of the volumetric flask, add 60% ethyl alcohol to 5. 0ml. Add 60% of the ethyl alcohol to 5. 0ml, add 0. 3ml of sodium nitrate solution (10%) accurately, shake up. Six minutes later, add 0. 3ml of aluminium nitrate (10%) again, shake up. After laying 6minutes, add 4ml of sodium hydroxide (1mol/L) and diluted to the volume with distilled water, mix well, and allow to stang for 15minutes. Vacancy solution: suck 5. 0ml of 60% ethyl alcohol accurately, add to a 10ml of the volumetric flask. Add 60% of the ethyl alcohol to 5. 0ml, add 0. 3ml of sodium nitrate solution (10%) accurately, shake up. Six minutes later, add 0. 3ml of aluminium nitrate (10%) again, shake up. After laying 6minutes, add 4ml of sodium hydroxide (1mol/L) and diluted to the volume with distilled water, mix well, and allow to stang for 15minutes. Determine the absorbance as above described method, and calculate the content of the total flavones.

Table 2 – 1   Assay of the total flavone

Sample	crude drug	stir – fired drug	Charred Crataegi Fructus	Crataegi Fructus charcoal
A				
Content(%)				

3. The assay of the total organic acid

Take about 1g of the fine powder, weigh accurately. Put into 100ml of water, accurately measured, soaking for 4 hours with occasional shaking, and filter. Take 25ml of the filtrate, measured accurately, add 50ml of water, 2 drops of phenolphthalein, titrate with sodium hydroxide (0. 1ml/L) is equivalent to 6. 404mg of citric acid($C_6H_8O_7$). Calculated total organic acid as citric acid.

Table 2 –2   Assay of the total organic acid

Sample	crude drug	stir – fired drug	Charred Crataegi Fructus	Crataegi Fructus charcoal
Content(%)				

Experimental records

(1)Record the assay of the total flavones and the assay of the total organic acid experimental result, fill in the table 2 – 1 and table 2 – 2, respectively .

(2)Make a record of the problemsappeard during the experiment and explain the causes of the problems.

Matters needing attention

(1)Crataegi Fructus should be eliminated foreign matter and fallen kernels according to the " Pharmacopoeia of the People's Republic of China ".

(2)Distributing the standard of quality of stir – frying to yellow, stir – frying to brown and stir – frying to charcoal Crataegi Fructus.

(3)9100 – spectrophotometer should be preheated.

Questions

(1)Why Crataegi Fructus should be processed before use?

(2)What problem should you note when processing Crataegi Fructus? How to control the fire and standard of process?

(3)Which kind of compound do the organic acid and flavone belong to?

(4)What other methods can we use to determine their content of different processed products of Fructus Crataegi?

Related materials

Fructus Crataegi is the dried ripe fruit of *Crataegus pinnatifida* Bge. var major N. E. Br. , or *Crataegus pinnatifida* Bge. . Crataegi Fructus has the function of stimulating digestion and promote the functional activity of the stomach; improving the normal flow of qi and dissipate blood stasis. According to the theory of traditional Chinese medicine, the Crataegi Fructus has the different function through different processing, for instance, charred Crataegi Fructus shine in digeation and charcoal of Crataegi Fructus shine in convergence and homeostasis.

Modern study showed that the flavone and organic acid of charred Crataegi Fructus possess multifarious pharmacological action. The organic acid can strengthen the digestive enzymatic secernent of stomach, and can promote digestion. Crataegi Fructus also can intensify the activity of the gastric lipase and peptidase, for example, ursolic acid. The flavones has notable function to cure the cardiovascular disease, it can expand blood vessel, dramatic cardiotonic, decrease blood pressure and so on, for example, hyperoside and vitexin (Compound structure as shown in Fig. 2 – 1).

Hyperoside

vitexin

ursolic acid

实验三　槐米及槐米炭中鞣质的含量测定

【实验目的】

1. 了解槐米炒炭的目的意义。

2. 通过对槐米和槐米炭中鞣质的含量测定，验证"炒炭存性"的传统理论，进一步明确炒炭止血作用增强的原理。

【实验原理】

中药槐米具有凉血、止血功效，用于吐血、衄血、便血、崩漏和痔疮出血等，主含芦丁、三萜皂苷及鞣质。其中鞣质具有收敛、固涩、止血、止痢及抗菌消炎作用。

中医药传统理论认为，槐米炒炭能缓和其寒性，产生涩性，增强止血作用；现代化学及药理研究证实槐米炒炭后鞣质含量增高，止血作用明显增强。本实验采用干酪素法及比色法测定槐米中鞣质的含量。

【实验器材】

温度计（300℃），电炒锅，真空干烘箱，乳钵，烘箱，100ml 容量瓶，1ml、5ml×2、10ml 吸量管，10ml 棕色容量瓶×6（5 个用于标准曲线），100ml 圆底烧瓶，100ml 容电瓶，250ml 容量瓶，50ml 棕色容量瓶，振荡器，量筒，9100 - 分光光度计，冷凝器；醋酸、醋酸钠、干酪素碳酸钠、鞣酸、钨酸钠、磷酸、甲醇、槐米、槐米炭。

【实验内容】

1. 炮制方法

（1）生槐米 取原药材，除去杂质，筛去灰屑及枝梗。

（2）槐米炭 取净槐米，用中火炒至棕褐色，立即出锅，摊开，放凉。

2. 鞣质含量测定（干酪素法）

（1）标准曲线的制备 取经 80℃ 干燥 2 小时的鞣酸，精密称定，配制 0.1mg/1ml 的 30% 甲醇溶液。精确吸取 1.0、2.0、3.0、4.0、5.0ml 分别置于 10ml 棕色容量瓶中，加 30% 甲醇至 5.0ml，加 pH 5.0 醋酸 - 醋酸钠缓冲溶液至刻度，摇匀。精密吸取上述各溶液 1.0ml，分别置于 10ml 棕色容量瓶中，各加 Folin 试剂 0.5ml，混匀，再加 5% 碳酸钠溶液至刻度，摇匀。于空温放置 20 分钟后，以蒸馏水做空白，在 720nm 处测定吸收度，以吸收度为纵坐标，浓度为横坐标绘制标准曲线。

（2）样品液制及测定 精密称取槐米及炒炭槐米粗粉各 0.4g，置 100ml 测定烧瓶中加 30% 甲醇 30ml，回流提取 1 小时，药渣加 30% 甲醇 20ml 提取 2 次，每次 30 分钟，过滤于 100ml 容量瓶中，以 30% 甲醇洗涤药渣 3 次，每次 5ml，洗液与滤液合并，以 30% 甲醇稀释至刻度。

精密吸取上述滤液 3ml，置 25ml 容量瓶中，加 pH 5.0 的醋酸 - 醋酸钠缓冲溶液 10ml，30% 甲醇 7ml，混匀［溶液（1）］。

精密吸取 10ml 溶液（1），置已盛有于酪素 250mg 的 50ml 棕色容量瓶中，振荡 1 小时，然后过滤，滤液摇匀［溶液（2）］。

分别吸取溶液（1）和溶液（2）各 1.0ml，各置于 10ml 棕色容量瓶中，各加 Folin 试剂 0.5ml，混匀，再加 5% 碳酸钠溶液至刻度，摇匀。于室温放置 20 分钟后，以蒸馏水做空白，在 720nm 处测定吸收度，测得吸收度为 A1 和 A2，依两吸光度之差，求出鞣质量，计算出样品中的含量。

计算式：

$$含量 = \frac{C \cdot T}{W \cdot 1000} \times 100\%$$

式中，C 为由回归方程得到的鞣质量；T 为稀释度；W 为样品的重量。

表3-1　鞣质含量测定

样品	W（g）	A₁（ml）	A₂（ml）	A₁－A₂（ml）	C（μg/ml）	X（%）
生槐米						
槐米炭						

【实验记录】

（1）记录鞣质含量测定结果。

（2）记录实验中出现的问题并说明原因。

【注意事项】

（1）槐米炒炭时，铁锅温度不能超过250℃，槐米温度不能超过210℃。出炭率不能低82%。

（2）槐米干燥温度应不超过60℃。

【思考题】

（1）槐米主要止血成分是什么？

（2）炒时温度升高，鞣质含量多，止血作用增强。因此可以认为制炭时温度越高越好，对吗？为什么？

【相关资料】

槐米是豆科植物槐 *Sophora japonica* L. 的干燥花蕾，为凉血、止血药，用于吐血、血、便血、崩漏和痔疮出血等，为中医常用止血药，主含芦丁（rutin）、少量三萜皂苷，水解后得白桦脂醇（betulin）、槐二醇（sophoradiol）、葡萄糖、葡萄糖醛酸，另总鞣质。其中鞣质具有收敛、固涩、止血、止痢及抗菌消炎作用。

Experiment 3　The Assay of the Content of Tannin in Different Product of Sophorae Flos

Purpose

1. To master the processing method of Sophorae Flos.

2. To understand the effect of processing on Sophorae Flos through the comparison of the content of tannin.

Prinliple

Sophorae Flos has the function which can arrest the bleeding by reducing the heat in blood. It is often used in the cases of hematochezia, hemorrhoidal bleeding, dysentery with bloody stools, abnormal uterine bleeding, spitting of blood and epistaxis. It contains rutin and triterpenic saponin which can become betulin, sophoradiol, glucose and half aldehyde.

Sophorae Flos also contains tannin which has the function of astringing, including astringency, arresting bleeding, antisepsis and arresting dysentery. According to the principle of traditional Chinese medicine, carbonizing can alleviate the nature of Sophorae Flos, produce the astringrncy and then strengthen the effect of arresting bleeding. The modern chemical and pharmacological studies have confirmed that the content of tannin has been increased after carbonizing. This conclusion will be showed in the experiment.

This experiment uses the method of potassium permanganate method, cheese method to determine the content oftannin.

Instruments and chemicals

1. Instruments

9100 – spectrophotometer, pot, iron shovel, enamel plate, the pot of water bath, analytical balance, volumetric flask (10ml, 25ml, 100ml), 10ml amber volumetric flask, measuring cylinder (10ml, 100ml, 500ml), 100ml round bottom beaker, 10ml suction pipet, acid buret (5ml, 10ml, 25ml), fitter paper, glass rod, separating funnel, beaker, electric furnace, incipient fusion glass funnel, thermometer.

2. Chemicals

Sophorae Flos, tannic acid (CRS), $KMnO_4$, concentrated sulfuric acid, indicarmine, NaCl, BaSO4, gelatin, acetate, sodium acetate, cheese, sodium carbonate, tannic acid, sodium tungstate, sodium nitrite, aluminium nitrate, sodium hydrate, methanol(AR), ether (AR).

Experimental content

1. Processing

Sophorae Flos: Eliminate the impurities and grey chip.

Sophorae Flos(Stir – frying to charcoal): Put the clean Sophorae Flos Immaturus in hot pot, heat with medium heating fire, stir continuously until the drugs becomes focal brown.

2. The assay of the content of tannin inFlos Sophorae and its processed products The method of cheese

(1)Preparation of reference solution: Take tannic acid (CRS) previously, measure accurately, put in vacuum to constant weight at 80℃ for 2 hours to prepare the 30% methanol solution containing 0.1mg/1ml tannic acid. Measure accurately 1.0, 2.0, 3.0, 4.0 and 5.0ml, respectively, into 10ml amber volumetric flask. Add 30% methanol to 5.0ml, and add pH5.0 acetic acid – sodium acetate butter to volume and mix well.

Measure 10ml of above – mentioned solution accurately into 10ml amber volumetric flask. Add respectively 0.5ml of Folin regent, mix well, add 5% sodium carbonate solution to volume and mix well. Allow to stand for 20 minutes and measure the absorbance at 720nm taking distilled water as vacancy. Take the absorbance as ordinate and the concentration as absorbance and plot the standard curve.

(2)Preparation of test solution: Take 0.4g of Sophorae Flos and Sophorae Flos carbonizing, respectively, weigh accurately, add into 100ml round bottom flask, add 30ml methanol to extract for 1 hour, filter. Extract the residue with 20ml methanol for 2 times, 30minutes per time. Filter into a 100ml volumetric flask and wash the residue with 5ml of 30% methanol for

3 times. Combine the washings into the flask and add 30% methanol to volume.

Measure 3ml of the above – mentioned solutions accurately into 25ml volumetric flask;add 10ml of pH5. 0 acetic acid – sodium acetate buffer and 7ml of 30% methanol to volume. Mix well and record as solution(1).

Measure accurately 10ml of the solutions into a 50ml amber volumetric flask,containing 250mg cheese and shake in the oscillating instrument for 1 hour. Filter and mix well and record as solution(2).

(3)Assay of tannic acid:Measure accurately 10ml of solution (1) and solution (2) into 10ml amber volumetric flask. Add respectively 0. 5ml of Folin regent,mix well,add 5% sodium carbonate solution to volume and mix well. Allow to stand for 20 minutes and measure the absorbance at 720nm taking distilled water as vacancy. Measure the absorbance A1 and A2 and calculate the content of tannin on the base of difference of A1 and A2.

$$X\% = \frac{C \cdot T}{W \cdot 1000} \times 100\%$$

X—the content of tannin (%)

C—the concentration of the test solution (μg/ml)

T—the dilution

W—the weigh of the sample(g)

Table 3 – 1   The assaying of the content of tannin (The method of cheese)

Sample	W(g)	A_1(ml)	A_2(ml)	$A_1 - A_2$(ml)	C(μg/ml)	X(%)
Crude drug						
Processed drug						

Experimental records

1. Record the experimental result of the tannin content in Flos Sophorae and its processed products,fill in the table 3 – 1.

2. Make a record of the problems appeard during the experiment and explain the causes of the problems.

Matters needing attention

1. The temperature of the pot should be not more than 250℃ and the temperature of the Flos Sophorae should be not more than 210℃. Eliminate the impurities and grey chip completely before weighing. Calculate the carbonation rate. The carbonation rate should be not less than 82%.

2. Sophorae Flos should be dried at temperature of 60℃.

Questions

1. Which chemical components can arrest the bleeding?

2. The temperature is higher,the content of tannin is higher and the effect of arresting the bleeding is strengthened. Can we think that temperature is higher,the result is better?

Related materials

Sophorae Flos is the dried flower bud of *Sophora japonica* L. It can arrest the bleeding by reducing the heat in blood. It is often used for hematochezia, hemorrhoidal bleeding, dysentery with bloody stools, abnormal uterine bleeding, spitting of blood and epistaxis. It contains rutin and triterpenic saponin which can become betulin, sophoradiol, glucose and half aldehyde.

实验四　加固体辅料炒法

【实验目的】

1. 掌握加固体辅料炒的方法及质量标准。
2. 掌握加固体辅料炒的火候及注意事项。
3. 了解加固体辅料炒的目的和意义。

【实验原理】

炒法分清炒和加辅料炒两种。根据辅料的不同，加辅料炒分为麸炒、米炒、土炒、砂炒、蛤粉炒、滑石粉炒。加辅料炒多用"中火"，砂炒多用"武火"。炒制的目的是为了改变药性，提高疗效，降低毒性和减少副作用，矫味、矫臭及便于制剂等。

【实验器材】

炉子、锅、铁铲、筛子、台秤、瓷盆、温度计等。

【实验内容】

一、麸炒

1. **苍术**　先将麦麸撒于热锅内，用中火加热，至冒烟时，加入苍术片，翻炒至表面深黄色，取出。筛去麦麸，放凉。

每100kg苍术片，用麦麸10kg。

成品性状：本品表面呈深黄色。有香气。

2. **枳壳**　先将麦麸撒于热锅内，用中火加热，至冒烟时倒入枳壳片，迅速翻动，炒至枳壳表面淡黄色时，取出。筛去麦麸，放凉。

每100kg枳壳片，用麦麸10kg。

成品性状：本品呈淡黄色。具香气。

3. **僵蚕**　先将麦麸撒于热锅内，用中火加热，至冒烟时，加入净僵蚕，翻炒至表面黄色，取出。筛去麦麸，放凉。

每100kg僵蚕，用麦麸10kg。

成品性状：本品表面呈淡黄色至黄色。腥气较微弱。

二、米炒

1. **斑蝥**　取净斑蝥与米置热锅内，用中火加热，翻炒至米呈黄棕色，取出。筛去米粒，放凉。

每 100kg 斑蝥，用大米 20kg。

成品性状：本品微挂火色。臭气轻微。

2. 党参 将大米置热锅内，用中火加热，至大米冒烟时，倒入党参片，翻炒至大米呈焦褐色，党参呈老黄色时，取出。筛去米，放凉。

每 100kg 党参片，用大米 20kg。

成品性状：本品表面呈老黄色，微有褐色斑点。具香气。

三、土炒

1. 山药 先将灶心土（或黄土，或赤石脂）置热锅内，用中火加热，至土粉呈灵活状态时，倒入山药片，不断翻炒，至山药挂土色，表面显土黄色，并透出山药固有香气时，取出。筛去土，放凉。

每 100kg 山药，用土 30kg。

成品性状：本品表面轻挂薄土，呈土黄色，无焦黑斑和焦苦味。具土香气。

2. 白术 先将灶心土（或黄土，或赤石脂）置热锅内，用中火加热，至土粉呈灵活状态时，倒入白术片，不断翻炒至外表挂有土色，并透出山药固有香气时，取出。筛去土，放凉。

每 100kg 白术，用土 30kg。

成品性状：本品表面呈土黄色，无焦黑斑和焦苦味。具土香气。

四、砂烫

1. 骨碎补 取净河砂，武火炒至滑利，投入骨碎补片（大小分档），不断翻动，炒至鼓起，取出，筛去砂，放凉，撞去毛。

成品性状：本品砂炒后为扁圆状鼓起，质轻脆，表面棕褐色或焦黄色，无鳞叶，断面淡棕褐色或淡棕色，味微涩，气香。

2. 穿山甲 将净砂置热锅内，用武火加热，至滑利容易翻动时，倒入大小一致的穿山甲片，不断翻炒，至鼓起，表面呈金黄色，边缘向内卷曲时，取出。筛去砂子，及时倒入醋中，搅拌，稍浸，捞出，干燥。

每 100kg 穿山甲，用米醋 30kg。

成品性状：本品膨胀鼓起，边缘向内卷曲，表面金黄色，质脆。略有醋气。

3. 鸡内金 将净砂置热锅内，用中火加热，至滑利容易翻动时，倒入大小一致的鸡内金，不断翻炒，至鼓起，卷曲，表面金黄色时，立即取出。筛去砂，放凉。

成品性状：本品膨胀鼓起，表面金黄色，质脆。具焦香气。

4. 马钱子 将净砂置热锅内，用武火加热，至滑利容易翻动时，投入马钱子，不断翻炒，至外表呈棕褐色或深褐色，内部鼓起小泡时，取出。筛去砂，放凉。

成品性状：本品表面呈深褐色或褐色，击之易碎，其内面鼓起小泡。具苦香味。

五、蛤粉烫

阿胶 先将胶块烘软，切成边长 10mm 的小胶丁备用。

取蛤粉置热锅内，用中火加热至灵活状态，放入阿胶丁，不断翻埋，烫至阿胶丁鼓起呈圆球形，内无"溏心"，颜色由乌黑转为深黄色，表面附着一层薄薄的蛤粉时，迅速取出。筛去蛤粉，放凉。

每100kg阿胶，用蛤粉40kg。

成品性状：本品呈类圆球形，表面灰白色至灰褐色，内无"溏心"，质轻而脆，中空，略成海绵状。

六、滑石粉烫

水蛭　先将滑石粉置热锅内，用中火加热至灵活状态，倒入净水蛭段，勤翻炒至微鼓起，呈黄棕色时取出。筛去滑石粉，放凉。

成品性状：本品淡黄色或黄棕色，微鼓起，质松脆，易碎。有腥气。

【实验记录】

（1）记录加辅料炒中各种药物形态、颜色、气味的变化。

（2）记录实验中出现的问题并说明原因。

【注意事项】

（1）加辅料炒制的药材炒制前应按照大小分档，避免受热不均，根据要求控制火力、火候。

（2）加辅料炒操作过程中，要勤翻动，使药物受热均匀，避免生熟不均的现象。

【思考题】

（1）实验药物加入固体辅料炮制的目的是什么？

（2）烫制药物为什么要掌握适当的温度，过高过低对药物有何影响？

（3）为什么严格控制辅料的用量？

Experiment 4　Stir – frying with Solid Adjuvant

Purpose

1. To master the processing method and quality standard of stir – frying drugs with solid adjuvant.

2. To master the heating strength and degree of stir – frying drugs with solid adjuvant, to master the matters need attention.

3. To understand the processing purpose of stir – frying drugs with solid adjuvant.

Principle

The processing methods of stir – frying drugs in a caldron include stir – frying drugs without adjuvant and stir – frying with solid adjuvant. According to different adjuvant of using, the processing method of stir – frying drugs with solid adjuvant include stir – frying with bran, stir – frying with rice, stir – frying with oven earth, stir – frying with sand, stir – frying with pulverized – clamshell, and stir – frying with pulverized – talcum.

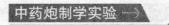

The purposes of stir – frying drugs with solid adjuvant can be briefly summarized as follows, removing or reducing the toxicity, promoting therapeutic effects; Take away the impurity, non – pharmaceutical parts and unpleasant tastes, drastic properties and side – effects of some Chinese medicinal herbs.

Instruments

Pot, stove, shovel, ceramic bowl, sieve, thermometer, balance, etc. .

Experimental Contents

1. Stir – frying with wheat bran

(1) Atractylodis Rhizoma (Cangzhu): Rhizoma Atractylodis stir – fried with wheat bran: Preheat the pot. Spread wheat bran into the hot pot evenly. Put the clean Rhizoma Atractylodis slice in hot pot while the smoke rises. Stir – frying with medium heating fire until the drugs becomes dark yellow. Sift out wheat bran. Chill before serving.

Every 100kg of Rhizoma Atractylodis, use 10kg of wheat bran.

(2) Aurantii Fructus (Zhiqiao): Aurantii Fructus stir – fried with wheat bran: Preheat the pot. Spread wheat bran into the hot pot evenly. Put the clean Aurantii Fructus slice in hot pot while the smoke rises. Stir – frying with medium heating fire until the drugs becomes pale yellow . Sift out wheat bran. Chill before serving.

Every 100kg of Fructus Aurantii, use 10kg of wheat bran.

(3) Bombyx Batryticatus (Jiangcan): Bombyx Batryticatus stir – fried with wheat bran: Preheat the pot. Spread wheat bran into the hot pot evenly. Put the clean Bombyx Batryticatus in hot pot while the smoke rises. Stir – frying with medium heating fire until the drugs becomes yellow. Sift out wheat bran. Chill before serving.

Every 100kg of Bombyx Batryticatus, use 10kg of wheat bran.

2. Stir – frying with rice

(1) Mylabris (Banmao): Mylabris stir – fried with rice: Preheat the pot. Spread rice into the hot pot evenly. Put the clean Mylabris in hot pot while the smoke rises. Stir – frying with medium heating fire until the rice becomes dark yellow. Sift out rice. Chill before serving.

Every 100kg of Mylabris, use 20kg of rice.

(2) Codonopsis Radix (Dangshen): Codonopsis Radix stir – fried with rice: Preheat the pot. Spread rice into the hot pot evenly. Put the clean Codonopsis Radix slice in hot pot while the smoke rises. Stir – frying with medium heating fire until the drugs becomes dark yellow. Sift out rice. Chill before serving.

Every 100kg of Codonopsis Radix, use 20kg of rice.

3. Stir – frying with oven earth

(1) Dioscoreae Rhizoma (Shanyao): Dioscoreae Rhizoma stir – fried with oven earth: Preheat the pot. Put oven earth into the hot pot evenly and heat it. . Put the clean Rhizoma Dioscorea slice in pot as soon as the oven earth becomes smooth. Stir – frying with medium heating fire until the drugs becomes earthy yellow and thesurface are covered by a layer of earth

powder evenly. Sift out oven earth. Chill before serving.

Every 100kg of Rhizoma Dioscoreae, use 30kg of oven earth.

(2) Rhizoma Atractylodis (Baizhu): Rhizoma Atractylodis stir – fried with oven earth: Preheat the pot. Put oven earth into the hot pot evenly and heat it. Put the clean Rhizoma Atractylodis slice in pot as soon as the oven earth becomes smooth. Stir – frying with medium heating fire until the drugs becomes earthy yellow and surface of the drugs are covered by a layer of earth powder evenly. Sift out oven earth. Chill before serving.

Every 100kg of Rhizoma Atractylodis, use 30kg of oven earth.

4. Stir – frying with sand

(1) Drynariae Rhizoma (Gusuibu): Drynariae Rhizoma stir – fried with sand: Put sand in the pot and heat it with strong heating fire until the sand becomes smooth. Put the clean Drynariae Rhizoma in pot. Stir – frying until the drugs becomes swell. Sift out the sand and remove the fuzz. Chill before serving.

Every 100kg of Drynariae Rhizoma, use 30kg of sand.

(2) Manis Squama (Chuanshanjia): Manis Squama stir – fried with sand: Put sand in the pot and heat it with strong heating fire until the sand becomes smooth. Put the clean Manis Squama with even size in pot. Stir – frying until the surface of drugs occur golden yellow and the whole part expand and curve inwardly. Sift out sand. Chill before serving. Or immerse the drugs in vinegar while they are hot. Remove out from the vinegar. Dry it.

Every 100kg of Manis Squama, use 30kg of sand.

(3) Galli Gigerii Endothlium (Jineijin): Galli Gigerii Endothlium stir – fried with sand: Put sand in the pot and heat it with strong heating fire until the sand becomes smooth. Put the clean Galli Gigerii Endothlium with even size in pot. Stir – frying until the surface of drugs occur golden yellow and the whole part expand and curve inwardly. Sift out sand. Chill before serving.

Every 100kg of Galli Gigerii Endothlium, use 30kg of sand.

(4) Strychni Semen (Maqianzi): Strychni Semen stir – fried with sand: Put sand in the pot and heat it with strong heating fire until the sand becomes smooth. Put the clean Semen Strychni with even size in pot. Stir – frying until the surface of drugs occur dark brown and the inner part bulges like bubble. Sift out sand and remove the fuzz. Chill before serving.

Every 100kg of Strychni Semen, use 30kg of sand.

5. Stir – frying with pulverized – clamshell

Asini Corii Colla: Bake the Asini Corii Colla with mild fire to make it soft. Cut it into small cubes.

Asini Corii Colla Stir – fried with pulverized – clamshell: Put pulverized – clamshell in the pot and heat it with strong heating fire until the pulverized – clamshell becomes smooth. Put the clean Asini Corii Colla cubes with even size in pot. Stir – frying until the whole part of Colla Corii Asini expand to become spherical without soft yolk core. Sift out pulverized – clamshell.

Chill before serving.

Every 100kg of Colla Corii Asini, use 40kg of pulverized – clamshell.

6. Stir – frying with pulverized – talcum

Hirudo（Shuizhi）：

Hirudo stir – fried with pulverized – talcum：Put pulverized – talcum in the pot and heat it with medium heating fire until the pulverized – talcum becomes smooth. Put the clean Hirudo with even size in pot. Stir – frying until surface of the drugs occur yellowish – brown and the whole part expand. Sift out pulverized – talcum. Chill before serving.

Every 100kg of Hirudo, use 40kg of pulverized – talcum.

Experimental records

1. Record the changes of form, color and odour during the processing of stir – frying drugs with solid adjuvant.

2. Make a record of the problems appeard during the experiment and explain the causes of the problems.

Matters needing attention

1. Separate the crude drugs by size before stir – frying, avoid uneven heating. During the processing, stir – fry the drug with solid adjuvant at appropriate temperature.

2. During the process of stir – frying the drug with solid adjuvant, it is necessary to stir frequently in order that the drugs is heated evenly, avoid uneven heated.

Reflection Questions

1. What is the main purpose of stir – frying drugs with solid adjuvant?

2. Why should we master the proper temperature of stir – frying drugs with solid adjuvant?

3. Why should we control adjuvant consumption strictly?

实验五　生枳壳与麸炒枳壳中总挥发油的含量及薄层鉴别比较

【实验目的】

1. 掌握麸炒枳壳的炮制方法，火候及注意事项。

2. 掌握挥发油含量测定法。通过枳壳麸炒炮制前后挥发油的比较，以及薄层鉴别比较，了解枳壳炮制的目的和意义。

3. 了解麸炒的目的和意义。

【实验原理】

枳壳来源于芸香科植物酸橙 *Citrus aurantium* L. 及其栽培变种的干燥未成熟果实。7月份果皮尚绿时采收，自中部横切为两半，晒干或低温干燥。本品性温，味苦、辛、酸。归脾、胃经。生枳壳辛燥，作用较强，偏于行气宽中消胀。用于气实壅满所致之脘腹胀痛或胁肋胀痛，瘀滞疼痛；子宫脱垂，脱肛，胃下垂。麸炒后减低其刺激性，缓和燥性和酸性，增强健脾消胀作用。麸炒枳壳因其作用缓和，而适宜于年老体弱而气滞者。

实验采用挥发油测定器，对枳壳麸炒前后枳壳中总挥发油的含量进行测定，同时，对麸炒前后枳壳进行薄层鉴别比较，进而说明麸炒炮制的意义。

【实验器材】

1. **仪器** 炒锅、铁铲、漏勺、液化气、分析天平、烧杯、圆底烧瓶、挥发油测定器、量筒、比重计、电炉、枳壳、麦麸、层析缸、玻璃板、硅胶、毛细管、烘箱等。

2. **试剂** 乙酸乙酯、甲醇、冰醋酸、硫酸、乙醇等。

【实验内容】

1. **药材的炮制**

（1）枳壳 取原药材，除去杂质，洗净，润透，去瓤，切薄片，干燥，筛去碎落的瓤核。

（2）麸炒枳壳 先将锅烧热，均匀撒入定量的麦麸，用中火加热，待烟起投入枳壳片，快速翻动，炒至淡黄色时取出，筛去麦麸，放凉。

每 100kg 枳壳片，用麦麸 10kg。

2. **总挥发油含量测定** 取生枳壳及麸炒枳壳粉末（过 2～3 号筛）各 40g 精密称定，分别置于 1000ml 烧瓶中，加水适量（约 300～400ml），集碎瓷片数片，混合，振摇，连接挥发油测定器与冷凝管。自冷凝管上端加水直至使其充满挥发油测定器的刻度部分，并溢流入烧瓶为止。置电热套上加热至沸，并保持微沸 3～4 小时，至测定器中油量不再增加时停止加热。放置片刻，开启测定器下端的活塞，将水缓缓放出，至油层上端到达 0 刻度线以上约 5mm 处。放冷，再开启活塞使油层下降至其上端恰与刻度 0 线平齐，读取挥发油量，并计算供试品中挥发油中的含量（%）。填入表 5-1。

表 5-1 总挥发油含量测定数据表

样品	挥发油含量（ml）
生枳壳	
麸炒枳壳	

3. **枳壳生品和制品的薄层鉴别比较** 取枳壳生品和制品粉末各 1g，分别置具塞试管中，加甲醇 5ml，密塞，超声提取 30 分钟，静置，取上清液作为供试品溶液。取生品和制品的供试品溶液等量，分别点于同一硅胶 G 薄层板上，乙酸乙酯-甲醇-冰醋酸（15:2:1）展开，取出晾干，先于紫外光灯（365nm）下检视，后喷以 10% 硫酸乙醇试剂，加热至斑点显色清晰（或喷以 $FeCl_3$/铁氰化钾试剂至斑点显色清晰）。比较枳壳生品和制品的斑点个数、大小、颜色深浅，讨论炮制对于枳壳化学成分的影响。

【实验记录】

（1）记录总挥发油含量测定数据，填入表 5-1。

（2）记录生品和制品的薄层鉴别比较结果。

（3）记录实验中出现的问题并说明原因。

【注意事项】

（1）枳壳生品和制品的薄层鉴别比较中，要仔细观察斑点大小、颜色深浅。

（2）在读取挥发油量时，应静置一段时间，使其充分与水分层。

（3）比重管须恒重。

（4）挥发油在测定其物理常数前，应脱水处理。

【思考题】

（1）根据你所查阅的文献，谈谈枳壳炮制前后药理作用有何变化？

（2）枳壳的炮制原理是什么？

【相关资料】

炮制对含挥发油类成分中药的影响如下。

挥发油大多具有芳香气味，常温下即可自行挥发而不留任何油迹。挥发油在水中溶解度极小，而易溶于有机溶剂。挥发油通常也是一种具有治疗作用的活性成分，在许多植物中含有挥发性的香气物质，要尽量保护，以免挥发油损失，对加热处理尤须注意，一般认为不可用火处理。含挥发性的药材应及时加工处理，干燥宜阴干。

相反，某些药物在炮制过程中，需要通过炮制以减少或除去挥发油，以除去某些挥发油的副作用，达到医疗的需要。如蜜炙麻黄，通过蜜炙加热处理，麻黄中具发汗作用的挥发油可减少，从而使所含的具有平喘作用的麻黄碱含量相对提高，再加上蜂蜜的协同作用，更适用于喘咳的治疗。蜜麻黄作用更缓和，适于表证已解而喘咳未愈的老人、幼儿及体虚患者。

另一方面，某些药物中的挥发油，具有毒性，如乳香，所含挥发油具有明显的毒性和强烈的刺激性，通过炮制后可大部分除去，有利临床应用。

Experiment 5　The Determination of Volatile Oil and TLC Analysis in Aurantii Fructus and Processed Products

Purpose

1. To master the processing of Aurantii Fructus.

2. To study the assay of volatile oil in Aurantii Fructus. To understand the processing purpose and meaning of stir – frying with wheat bran through the volatile oil content TLC assay of different processed products.

3. To understand the processing purpose of stir – frying with wheat bran.

Principle

Aurantii Fructus is origin from the dried, immature fruit of *Citeus aurantium* L. and its cultivated varieties. The property of Fructus Aurantii is warm, bitter, acrid and sour; attribution to the spleen and stomach channel. It has the function of regulating the flow of qi, removing its stagnation, and alleviating distension. The effect of crude Fructus Aurantii is stronger, can be used to eliminate stagnation of qi and relieve stuffiness sensation in the chest and abdomen. After stir – frying with wheat bran, its stimulation will lower, its dryness character and sour character will be mild and its effect of invigorating the spleen and relieve stuffiness sensation in chest and abdomen will be enhanced. Then the processed products is used for the old patients.

In this experiment, we will determine the content of volatile oil in crude drugs and processed products; TLC assay is also used to explain the meaning of processing.

Instruments and chemicals

1. Instruments

Pot, slice, strainer, gas, analytical balance, breaker, flask, volumetric oil determination apparatus, measuring cylinder, electricfurnace, gravimeter etc.

2. Chemicals

Ethyl acetate, methanol, glacial acetic acid, Fructus Aurantii, bran etc.

Experimental content

1. Processing

(1) Fructus Aurantii: Take crude Fructus Aurantii, eliminate impurities and grey chip, wash, soften thoroughly, cut into thin slices, dry, sift out the broken pulp and seeds.

(2) Fructus Aurantii stir – frying with wheat bran: Preheat the pot. Spread wheat bran into the hot pot evenly. Put the clean Fructus Aurantii slice in hot pot while the smoke rises. Stir – frying with medium heating fire until the drugs becomes pale yellow. Sift out wheat bran. Chill before serving.

Every 100kg of Fructus Aurantii, use 10kg of wheat bran.

2. Determination of volatile oil

Take 40g of crude drug and prepared drug powder, weigh accurately, add into flasks respectively. Add moderate water (about 300—400ml) and a few glass beads, shake and mix well. Connect flask to volatile oil determination tube and then connect to reflux condenser. Add water through the top of reflux consider until the graduated tube is filled and overflows to flask. Heat the flask gently in an electric heating jacket or by other suitable means until boiling begins, and continue heating for about 3—4 hours until the volume of oil does not increase. Stop heating, stand for a few minutes, and open the stopcock at lower, run off the water layer solely until the volatile oil layer is 5mm above the zero mark. Stand until it becomes cold, open the stopcock again, run off the remaining water layer carefully until the volatile oil layer is just on zero mark. Read the volume of oil in the graduated portion of the tube, and calculate the content of volatile oil.

Table 5 – 1　The content of volatile oil

Sample	The volatile oil (ml)
Crude drug	
Processed drug	

3. Comparison on different processed products of Fructus Aurantii by TLC method

Take the crude drug and processed product of Fructus Aurantii 1g into test tube respectively. Add 5ml methyl alcohol, dense plug, extracted with ultrasonic for 30 minutes, standing. Take the upper clear liquid as the test solution.

Take equivalent crude drug and processed product of Fructus Aurantii solution, point on the same silica G thin layer plate respectively. Use ethyl acetate - methanol - glacial acetic acid (15:2:1), as developing solvent. Take out to dry. Discuss the influence of the chemical composition because of processing according to the number, size and color of the spots.

Experimental records

(1) Record the content of volatile oil, fill in the table 5 - 1.

(2) Record the TLC results.

(3) Make a record of the problems appeared during the experiment and explain the causes of the problems.

Matters needing attention

(1) In the TLC experiment, the number, size and color of spots should be observed carefully.

(2) Waiting for a few minutes to allow the water layer separate thoroughly from the oily layer, when the volume of oil in the graduated portion of the tube is read.

(3) Pycnometer must be constant weight.

(4) Volatile oil should be dehydrated when determining its physical constant.

Reflection Questions

(1) Please study the change of pharmacological action after processing, through consult the reports

(2) What is the processing principle of Aurantii Fructus?

Related materials

The changes in traditional Chinese medicines containing volatile oil by processing.

Volatile oil has a fragrant smell, and can give off itself and doesn't have any oil marks under normal atmospheric temperatures. It is difficult to be dissolved into water and easy to be dissolved in the organic solvent. Volatile oil is a kind of components having bio - activity in traditional Chinese medicines. Most of traditional Chinese medicines have expelling superficial evils, relieving cough and having spicy flavour. Different processing method have different effects in the clinic of TCM. For example, the Chinese medicine contains essential oil which is effective components without side - effect. They must be dried in the shady place instead of the sunshine or on the fire.

Sometimes, traditional Chinese medicines contain volatile oil having certain side - effects, we need reduce their quantities of the oil by processing for clinical application, such as **Herba Ephedrae** (Mahuang). The origin Herba Ephedrae has higher quantities of volatile oil, its effects of inducing sweat and dispelling exogenous evils are stronger. So it is usually used for some patients who are attacked by wind and cold evils without sweat. Stir – frying with honey, Herba Ephedrae has less quantity of volatile oil and its efficacy of inducing sweat is not stronger than the origin drugs. So it may be used for some poor constitutional patients, old patients and children.

On the contrary, a few traditional Chinese medicines contain the volatile oil which have some irritation and toxicity, such as frankincense (Ruxiang). The experiments showed that its irritation and toxicity are reduced evidently after it had been fried with vinegar. The reason can be explained that the volatile oil reduce partly by stir – frying with vinegar.

实验六 炙 法

【实验目的】

1. 掌握各种炙法的操作方法、注意事项、成品规格、辅料选择和一般用量。
2. 了解各种炙法的目的意义。

【实验原理】

将净选或切制后的药物,加入一定量的液体辅料拌炒,使辅料逐渐渗入药物组织内部的炮制方法称为炙法。

药物吸收一定的辅料,经加热处理后,在性味、功效、作用趋向、归经和理化性质均能发生某些变化,起到降低毒性,抑制偏性,增强疗效,矫臭矫味,使有效成分易于溶出,从而最大限度地发挥疗效。

【实验器材】

炉子、锅铲、铁锅、瓷盘、量筒、筛子、温度计、天平等。

【实验内容】

一、酒炙

1. 川芎 取净川芎片,用黄酒拌匀,闷润至酒被吸尽后,置热锅内,用文火加热,炒至棕黄色,取出放凉。筛去碎屑。

川芎每 100kg,用黄酒 10kg。

成品性状:本品呈棕黄色,微有酒气。

2. 当归 取净当归片,用黄酒拌匀,闷润至酒被吸尽后,置热锅内,用文火炒至深黄色,取出放凉。

辅料用量:每 100kg 当归,用黄酒 10kg。

成品性状:本品酒炙后呈老黄色,略有焦斑,微具酒气。

炮制作用:本品酒炙后增强活血补血调经的功效。

二、醋炙

1. 香附 取净香附粒块或片,加米醋拌匀,闷润至透,置热锅内,用文火加热,炒至香附微挂火色,取出晾干。筛去碎屑。

香附每 100kg，用米醋 20kg。

成品性状：本品制后颜色加深，微挂火色，具醋气。

2. **柴胡** 取净柴胡，加米醋拌匀，闷润至透，置锅内文火炒干，至柴胡呈黄褐色时，取出放凉。

辅料用量：柴胡每 100kg，用米醋 20kg。

成品性状：本品醋炙后，呈黄褐色，质干脆，具醋气。

炮制作用：本品生品升散力强，清热解表；醋炙后，缓和升散之性，增强疏肝止痛的功效。

三、盐炙

1. **知母** 取净知母片置锅中，用文火微炒至变色，喷洒盐水，炒干，取出放凉。

辅料用量：每 100kg 知母，用盐 2kg（加 4~5 倍量水溶解）。

成品性状：本品盐炙后，颜色加深，略有咸味。

炮制作用：知母生品苦寒滑利，泻肺胃肾火，润肠；盐炙后引药入肾经，增强滋阴降火之功效。

2. **车前子** 取净车前子，置热锅内，用文火加热，炒至略有爆裂声，微鼓起时，喷入盐水，炒干后取出放凉。

车前子每 100kg，用食盐 2kg。

成品性状：本品鼓起，部分存裂隙。味微咸。

3. **杜仲** 取杜仲丝或块，加盐水拌匀，稍闷，待盐水被吸尽后，置炒制容器内，用中火炒至表面焦黑色，丝易断时，取出晾凉。筛去碎屑。

每 100kg 杜仲块或丝，用食盐 2kg。

成品性状：杜仲呈小方块或丝状。外表淡棕色或灰褐色，粗糙，内表面暗紫色，光滑。质脆，易折断，断面有细密、银白色、富弹性的橡胶丝相连。气微，味略苦。盐杜仲表面呈焦黑色，折断时橡胶丝弹性较差，略有咸味。

四、蜜炙

1. **甘草** 取炼蜜加适量开水稀释，加入净甘草片内拌匀，闷润，置热锅内，用文火加热，炒至表面棕黄色，不粘手时，取出放凉。筛去碎屑。

甘草每 100kg，用炼蜜 25kg。

成品性状：本品呈棕黄色，微有光泽。味甜，具焦香气。

2. **黄芪** 取净黄芪片，用炼蜜加适量沸水稀释，与黄芪拌匀，稍闷，置锅内文火炒至深黄色，不粘手时，取出放凉。

辅料用量：每 100kg 黄芪，用炼蜜 25kg。

成品性状：本品蜜炙后，呈深黄色，质较脆，略带黏性，味甘。

炮制作用：黄芪生品长于益卫固表，托毒生肌，利尿退肿；蜜炙后长于益气补中。

五、姜炙

厚朴 取净厚朴丝，加姜汁拌匀，闷润，至姜汁完全吸尽，置热锅内，不断翻动，用文火加热，炒干，取出，放凉。筛去碎屑。

厚朴每100kg，用生姜10kg（干姜用1/3）。

成品性状：本品色泽加深，具姜的辛辣气味。

六、油脂炙

淫羊藿 先将羊脂油置锅内，用文火加热，至全部熔化时，倒入净淫羊藿丝，炒至微黄色，油脂被吸尽，取出放凉。

淫羊藿每100kg，用炼羊脂油20kg。

成品性状：本品表面微黄色，润泽光亮，质脆。具油香气。

【实验记录】

（1）记录各种炙法中药物形态、颜色、气味的变化。

（2）记录实验中出现的问题并说明原因。

【注意事项】

（1）各炙法中采用先拌辅料后炒方法炒制的药，一定要闷润至辅料完全被吸尽或渗透到药物组织内部后，才可进行炒制。酒炙药物闷润时，容器要加盖密闭，以防酒迅速挥发。后加辅料炙的药物，辅料要均匀喷洒在药物上，不要沿锅壁加入，以免辅料迅速蒸发。

（2）若液体辅料用量较少，不易与药物拌匀时，可先加适量开水稀释后，再与药物拌润。

（3）在炙炒时，火力不可过大，多用文火，翻炒宜勤，一般炒至近干，颜色加深时，即可出锅摊晾。

【思考题】

（1）实验中各药炮制目的是什么？

（2）蜜炙、油炙、姜炙、盐炙法所用辅料如何制备？

（3）为什么车前子常采用先炒药后加辅料的方法？

Experiment 6　The Method of Stir – frying with Liquid Adjuvant

Purpose

1. To master the processing method, quality standard, matters needing attention, material selection and general dosage of stir – frying drugs with liquid adjuvant.

2. To understand the processing purpose of stir – frying drugs with liquid adjuvant.

Principle

The effect of stir – frying drugs with liquid adjuvant can be briefly summarized as follows, removing or reducing the toxicity, promoting therapeutic effects; Take away the impurity, non – pharmaceutical parts and unpleasant tastes, drastic properties and side – effects of some Chinese medicinal herbs, so as to maximize therapeutic results.

Instruments

Pot, stove, shovel, ceramic bowl, measuring cylinder sieve, thermometer, balance, etc. .

Experimental Contents

1. The method of stir – frying with wine

(1) Chuanxiong Rhizoma (Chuanxiong): Chuanxiong Rhizoma stir – frying with wine: Mix up the clean Chuanxiong Rhizoma slice and yellow rice or millet wine. Cover tightly and moisten them until the yellow rice or millet wine is absorbed thoroughtly. Put Chuanxiong Rhizoma in the pot and heat it with mild heating fire until the Chuanxiong Rhizoma becomes dark yellow. Take the drugs out from the pot. Chill before serving.

Every 100kg of Szechuan Lovage Rhizome, use 10kg of yellow rice or millet wine.

(2) Angelicae Sinensis Radix (Danggui): Angelicae Sinensis Radix stir – frying with wine:

Mix up the clean Angelicae Sinensis Radix slice and yellow rice or millet wine. Cover tightly and moisten them until the yellow rice or millet wine is absorbed thoroughtly. Put Angelicae Sinensis Radix in the pot and stir – fry with mild heating fire until the Angelicae Sinensis Radix becomes dark yellow. Take the drugs out from the pot. Chill before serving.

Every 100kg of Chinese angelica, use 10kg of yellow rice or millet wine.

2. The method of stir – frying with vinegar

(1) Cyperi Rhizoma (Xiangfu): Cyperi Rhizoma (Xiangfu) stir – frying with vinegar:

Mix up the clean Cyperi Rhizoma and rice vinegar. Cover tightly and moisten them until the rice vinegar is absorbed thoroughtly. Put Cyperi Rhizoma in the pot and stir – fry with mild heating fire until the Cyperi Rhizoma dry. Take the drugs out from the pot. Chill before serving.

Every 100kg of Cyperi Rhizoma, use 20kg of rice vinegar.

(2) Bupleuri Radix(Chaihu): Bupleuri Radix stir – frying with vinegar:

Mix up the clean Bupleuri Radix and rice vinegar. Cover tightly and moisten them until the rice vinegar is absorbed thoroughtly. Put Bupleuri Radix in the pot and stir – fry with mild heating fire until the Bupleuri Radix dry. Take the drugs out from the pot. Chill before serving.

Every 100kg of Bupleuri Radix, use 20kg of rice vinegar.

3. The method of stir – frying with salt

(1) Anemarrhenae Rhizoma (Zhimu)   Anemarrhenae Rhizoma stir – frying with salt: Put Anemarrhenae Rhizoma slice in the pot and stir – fry with mild heating fire until the color changes. Sprinkle a certain amount of salt water. Go on to stir – fry until the drugs dry. Take the drugs out from the pot. Chill before serving.

Every 100kg of Anemarrhenae Rhizoma, use 2kg of salt.

(2) Plantaginis Semen(Cheqianzi): Plantaginis Semen stir – frying with salt: Put Plantaginis Semen in the pot and stir – fry with mild heating fire until there is the sound of crack.

Sprinkle a certain amount of salt water. Go on to Stir – fry until the drugs dry. Take the drugs out from the pot. Chill before serving.

Every 100kg of Plantaginis Semen, use 2kg of salt.

（3）Eucommia Cortex（Duzhong）: Eucommia Cortex stir – frying with salt: Mix up the clean Eucommia Cortex and salt water. Cover tightly and moisten them until the salt water is absorbed thoroughly. Put Eucommia Cortex in the pot and stir – fry with mild heating fire until the color of Eucommia Cortex is darker with scorched spots and the thread is easy to be snapped. Take the drugs out from the pot. Chill before serving.

Every 100kg of Eucommia Cortex, use 2kg of salt.

4. The method of stir – frying with honey

（1）Glycyrrhizae Radix et Rhizoma（Gancao）: Glycyrrhizae Radix et Rhizoma stir – frying with honey: Mix up the clean Glycyrrhizae Radix et Rhizoma and honey. Cover tightly and moisten them until the honey is absorbed thoroughly. Put Glycyrrhizae Radix et Rhizoma in the pot and stir – fry with mild heating fire until the color of Glycyrrhizae Radix et Rhizoma is claybank and not glue the hand. Take the drugs out from the pot. Chill before serving.

Every 100kg of Glycyrrhizae Radix et Rhizoma, use 25kg of honey.

（2）Astragali Radix（Huangqi）: Astragali Radix stir – frying with honey: Mix up the clean Astragali Radix and honey. Cover tightly and moisten them until the honey is absorbed thoroughly. Put Astragali Radix in the pot and stir – fry with mild heating fire until the color of Astragali Radix is claybank and not glue the hand. Take the drugs out from the pot. Chill before serving.

Every 100kg of Astragali Radix, use 25kg of honey.

5. The method of stir – frying with ginger juice

Magnoliae Officinalis Cortex

Magnoliae Officinalis Cortex stir – frying with ginger juice: Mix up the clean Magnoliae Officinalis Cortex and ginger juice. Cover tightly and moisten them until the ginger juice is absorbed thoroughly. Put Magnoliae Officinalis Cortex in the pot and stir – fry with mild heating fire until the Magnoliae Officinalis Cortex dry. Take the drugs out from the pot. Chill before serving.

Every 100kg of Magnoliae Officinalis Cortex, use 10kg of ginger.

6. The method of Stir – frying with oil

Epimedii Folium（Yinyanghuo）

Epimedii Folium stir – frying with oil: Put sebum oil in the pot and stir – fry with mild heating fire to make it melt. Add the Epimedii Folium. Stir – fry with mild heating fire until the Epimedii Folium is slightly yellow, the oil is absorbed thoroughly. Take the drugs out from the pot. Chill before serving.

Every 100kg of Epimedii Folium, use 20kg of sebum oil.

Experimental records

(1) Record the changes ofform, color and odour during the processing of stir – frying with liquid adjuvant.

(2) Make a record of the problems appeard during the experiment and explain the causes of the problems.

Matters needing attention

(1) In the process of stir – frying with liquid adjuvant which mix the materials before stir – frying, you must moisten it until the liquid adjuvant was sufficiently absorbed by the crude drugs.

(2) If the dosage of liquid adjuvant is less, please add suitable amount of drinking water to dilute.

(3) Pay attention toheat power in the process of stir – frying with liquid adjuvant.

Reflection Questions

(1) What is the main purpose of the drugs stir – frying drugs with liquid adjuvant?

(2) How to prepare the adjuvant of stir – frying with wine, stir – frying with vinegar, stir – frying with salt, stir – frying with honey and stir – frying with ginger juice?

(3) Why do we stir – frying Semen plantaginis before adding saline water?

实验七　延胡索的炮制及炮制前后药理作用比较

【实验目的】

1. 掌握中药延胡索的炮制方法。

2. 通过对中药延胡索生品及醋制品药理作用的比较，说明延胡索的炮制作用。

【实验原理】

延胡索为罂粟科植物延胡索 *Corydalis yanhusuo* W. T. Wang 的干燥块茎。具有疏肝理气，行气止痛的作用。广泛用于治疗各种痛证。延胡索有多种炮制方法，一般以醋制为主。

醋制能加强延胡索疏肝止痛的作用。现代研究表明延胡索含生物碱类成分，其中延胡索乙素等叔胺型生物碱具有明显的止痛作用，是延胡索止痛的主要成分。醋制后，水煎剂中的总生物碱和延胡索乙素含量增加，从而止痛作用增强。本实验用小鼠进行镇痛试验，验证延胡索炮制作用。

【实验器材】

1. **仪器**　铁锅、铁铲、火炉、搪瓷盘、托盘天平、烧杯、量筒、水浴锅、电炉、灌胃器。

2. **试剂**　米醋、0.6%醋酸溶液等。

【实验内容】

一、药材的炮制

1. **延胡索** 取原药材，除去杂质，大小分开，洗净，稍浸、润透，切厚片，干燥。筛去碎屑；或洗净干燥后捣碎。

2. **醋延胡索** 取净延胡索或延胡索片，加入定量的米醋拌匀，闷润至醋被吸尽后，置炒制容器内，用文火加热，炒干，取出晾凉。筛去碎屑。

每100kg延胡索，用米醋20kg。

二、小鼠扭体镇痛试验

1. **样品液制备** 精密称取延胡索生品和制品各25g，分别置于1000ml烧杯中，用400ml和300ml水分别煎煮2次，每次保持微沸30分钟，用脱脂棉过滤，合并滤液，浓缩，以水定容于100ml容量瓶，备用。

2. **小鼠扭体镇痛试验** 取体重18~22g小鼠（雌雄各半）60只，随机分成3组，每组20只，分别灌胃给予生理盐水及上述样品液，每只0.6ml，剂量分别为7.5g生药/kg。40分钟后，腹腔注射0.6%醋酸溶液，剂量为0.1ml/10g，观察并记录10分钟内产生扭体反应的动物数，按公式计算镇痛百分率。

$$镇痛百分率 = \frac{N_1 - N_0}{N_2} \times 100\%$$

N_1：药物组无扭体反应的动物数

N_0：对照组无扭体反应的动物数

N_2：对照组扭体反应的动物数

表 7-1 镇痛百分率

样品	动物数	扭体反应数	镇痛百分率（%）
生延胡索			
醋延胡索			
生理盐水			

【实验记录】

（1）分别记录对照组、给药组扭体反应的小鼠数。

（2）记录实验中出现的问题并说明原因。

【注意事项】

（1）延胡索水煎液中有较多的黏液，可用脱脂棉过滤。

（2）小鼠体重差别不超过2g。

【思考题】

（1）延胡索为什么要炮制？

（2）通过对延胡索生品及醋制品止痛作用的差异，能得到什么结论？

Experiment 7 Comparative Studies on the Pharmaceutical Effects between the Crude and the Processed Drugs of Corydalis Rhizoma

Purpose

1. To master the processing method of Corydalis Rhizoma that stir – frying with vinegar.

2. To compare the pharmaceutical effects between the crude Corydalis Rhizoma and the processed products, to explain the processing action and processing principle.

Experimental principle

Rhizoma Corydlis is the dried tuber of *Corydalis yanhusuo* W. T. Wang. It can sooth the liver and regulate Qi. Rhizoma Corydlis can promote the flow of Qi and relieve the pain. According to the traditional Chinese medicine (TCM), it is used widely to relieve kinds of pains. There are many processing methods on Corydalis Rhizoma, but it is usually stir – fried with vinegar.

According to the principle of TCM, processing with rice vinegar for leading the drug effect into liver meridian, it can strengthen the drug's function about soothing the liver and releving paining. The processing with vinegar can increase Rhizoma Corydalis's function of relieving paining.

Modem studies showed that Corydalis Rhizoma mainly contains alkaloids, have the obviusly function of relieving pain. After stir – frying with vinegar, the amount of the total alkaloids were increased in the water extraction. As the result, the effect of relieving pain was increased.

Instruments and chemicals

1. Instruments

Pot, shovel, stove, enamel plate, table balance, baker, measuring cylinder, water bath kettle, electric stove, lavage apparatus.

2. Chemicals

Vinegar, 0.6% acetic acid.

Experimental content

1. The processing of crude drugs

(1) Corydalis Rhizoma: Take crude Rhizoma Corydalis, to eliminae impurities and grey chip, wash clean dry and break into pieces.

(2) Corydalis Rhizoma stir – frying with vinegar: Mix up the clean Corydalis Rhizoma and rice vinegar. Cover tightly and moisten them until the rice vinegar is absorbed thoroughtly. Put Corydalis Rhizoma in the pot and stir – fry with mild heating fire until the Corydalis Rhizoma dry. Take the drugs out from the pot. Chill before serving.

Every 100kg of Radix bupleuri, use 20kg of rice vinegar.

2. Writhing response and pain – relieving test on mice

(1) Preparation the sample: To weigh 25g of both the crude drug and the processed drug accurately. Put then into 1000ml beakers respectively 25g of both the crude brug and the pro-

cessed drug, then add 400ml and 300ml water to decoct the drug for two rimes. Each time, the decoction should keep slightly boiling for 30minutes. To filter the decoction with absorbent cotton then mix the filtrate and concentrated in the water bath, then transfer them to 100ml volumetric flask, then add water to dilute the each solution to graduation respecively.

（2）Writhing response and pain - relieving test on mice: To take 60 mice which weigh from 18g to 22g, and half of them are male, to divide the mice into four groups at random, each group has the same number. Given physiological saline and samples above mentioned to each group, the dose is 0.6ml/mouse; 40 minutes later, intraperitoneal injection 0.6% acetic acid with the dose of 0.1mg/10g, then observe and record the number of the mice which has distortion reacion within 10 minutes, then calculated through the following formula.

$$\text{The percentage of painrelieving} = \frac{N_1 - N_0}{N_2} \times 100\%$$

N_0: The number of mice which has no distortion reaction of the controlled group

N_1: The number of mice which has no distortion reaction of the drug given group

N_2: The number of mice which has distortion reaction of the controlled group

Table 7 - 1　The percentage of pain relieving

sample	Numbers of animal	Withing response number	The percentage of pain - relieving（%）
crude drug			
processed products			
Physiological Saline			

Experimental records

（1）Record the number of mice which has writhing response in the controlled group and the drug - given group respectively.

（2）Make a record of the problems appeard during the experiment and explain the causes of the problems.

Matters needing attention

The water decoction of Rhizoma Corydalis isn't easy to filtrate due to it has much starch, we can deal it with absorbent cotton.

Reflection Questions

1. Why we processed Rhizoma Corydalis?

2. Compare the percentage of pain - reliecing between the crude drug and processed drug, what can you conclude according to the variation?

实验八　延胡索炮制前后生物碱的含量测定

【实验目的】

通过对中药延胡索生品及醋制品中生物碱含量的测定，说明延胡索醋制的意义。

【实验原理】

延胡索为罂粟科植物延胡索 *Corydalis yanhusuo* W. T. Wang 的干燥块茎。具有疏肝理气、行气止痛的作用。临床广泛用于治疗各种痛证。

中医理论认为，醋能引药入肝，增强药物疏肝散瘀、止痛的功效。醋制能加强延胡索疏肝止痛的作用。现代研究表明延胡索含生物碱类成分，其中延胡索乙素等叔胺型生物碱具有明显的止痛作用，是延胡索止痛的主要成分。醋制后，水煎剂中的总生物碱和延胡索乙素（止痛有效成分）含量都会增加，从而止痛作用增强。本实验通过对延胡索醋制前后总生物碱的变化，说明延胡索炮制作用。

延胡索乙素

【实验器材】

1. 仪器 铁锅、铁铲、搪瓷盘、分析天平、称量瓶、烧杯、量筒、玻璃漏斗、分液漏斗、容量瓶、移液管、碱式滴定管。

2. 试剂 食醋、三氯甲烷（AR）、无水硫酸钠、0.01mol/L 硫酸、0.02mol/L 氢氧化钠、甲基红 – 溴甲酚绿指示剂等。

【实验内容】

一、药材的炮制

1. 延胡索 取原药材，除去杂质，大小分开，洗净，稍浸、润透，切厚片，干燥。筛去碎屑；或洗净干燥后捣碎。

2. 醋延胡索 取净延胡索或延胡索片，加入定量的米醋拌匀，闷润至醋被吸尽后，置炒制容器内，用文火加热，炒干，取出晾凉。筛去碎屑。

每 100kg 延胡索，用米醋 20kg。

二、总生物碱含量测定

1. 样品制备 精密称取延胡索生品和制品各 10g，分别置于 500ml 烧杯中，用 200ml 和 100ml 水分别煎煮 2 次，每次煎煮 30 分钟，用脱脂棉过滤，合并滤液，加氨水调至 pH10 以上，将滤液移至 250ml 分液漏斗中，用三氯甲烷萃取，至无生物碱反应。合并萃取液，用 20ml 蒸馏水洗涤，再用 5ml 三氯甲烷洗涤水层，合并三氯甲烷，加入 5g 无水硫酸钠脱水后，浓缩，转移至 10ml 容量瓶，以三氯甲烷定容至刻度。

2. 含量测定 精密吸取 5ml 上述样品，加入到 100ml 锥形瓶中，在通风橱内水浴挥干三氯甲烷，加 2ml 三氯甲烷溶解残渣，加 0.01mol/L 硫酸 20ml，在通风橱内水浴挥干三氯甲烷，用 0.2mol/L 的氢氧化钠溶液滴定，以甲基红 – 溴甲酚绿指示剂 2 滴，终点颜色由红变绿。根据公式计算总生物碱含量（按延胡索乙素计算）：

$$总生物碱含量（\%）=\frac{(N_{H_2SO_4}\cdot V_{H_2SO_4}-N_{NaOH}\cdot V_{NaOH})\times 355.4}{W\times 1000}\times D\times 100\%$$

（D：稀释度）

表 8 - 1　总生物碱含量

样品	重量（g）	NaOH 消耗量（ml）	总生物碱含量（%）
生延胡索			
醋延胡索			

【实验记录】

（1）记录延胡索生品和制品总生物碱含量测定结果，填入表 8 - 1。

（2）记录实验中出现的问题并说明原因。

【注意事项】

（1）三氯甲烷萃取要完全，以少量多次为佳；若三氯甲烷层乳化，可用玻棒搅拌助其分层。

（2）挥干三氯甲烷时，应在通风橱内，水浴挥干。

【思考题】

通过对延胡索生品及醋制品水煎液中总生物碱含量变化的比较，能得到什么结论？

【相关资料】

炮制对含生物碱类药物的影响如下。

生物碱是一类含氮的有机化合物，通常有似碱的性质，多数味苦，而且具有明显的生理活性。不但植物来源的中药可含有生物碱，而且动物来源的中药有的也含有生物碱（如蟾酥）。

1. 中药中含有游离生物碱　游离生物碱一般不溶或难溶于水，而能溶于乙醇、三氯甲烷等有机溶剂，亦可溶于酸水（形成盐），大多数生物碱盐类则可溶于水，难溶或不溶于有机溶媒，所以常用酒、醋等作为炮制辅料，以提高溶出度。酒既有极性溶媒的性质，又有非极性溶媒的性质，是一个良好的溶剂。中药化学成分的提取很多用醇，而酒就具有稀醇性质的溶剂。不论是游离生物碱或其盐类都能溶解。所以药物经过酒制后能提高生物碱的溶出率，从而提高药物的疗效。

醋是弱酸，能与游离生物碱结合成盐。生物碱的醋酸盐易被水溶出，增加水溶液中有效成分的含量，提高疗效。如延胡索主要的有效成分是延胡索乙素、延胡索甲素等，是具有止痛和镇静作用的生物碱，这两种生物碱以游离形式存在于植物中，难溶于水，但与醋酸结合生成乙酸盐，能溶于水，所以延胡索经醋制后，在水溶液中溶出量增加，从而增强了止痛效果。

生物碱在植物体中，也往往与植物体中的有机酸、无机酸生成复盐，如鞣酸盐、草酸盐等，他们是一种不溶于水的复盐，若加入醋酸后，可以取代上述复盐中的酸类，形成可溶于水的乙酸盐复盐，增加在水中的溶解度。

2. **中药中含有水溶性生物碱**　大多数生物碱不溶于水，但有些小分子生物碱如槟榔碱易溶于水，一些季铵类生物碱也能溶于水，在炮制过程中如用水洗、水浸等操作时，应尽量减少与水接触，在切制这类药材时，宜采取少泡多润的原则，尽量减少在切片浸泡过程中生物碱的损失，以免影响疗效。

3. **在不同药用部位，生物碱分布不同**　在植物不同部位，生物碱含量分布不同。钩藤过去常以双钩入药，现代药理证明茎枝降压程度与混钩无明显差异，生物碱含量一致。有实验表明，钩藤的钩与枝含有0.2%左右的生物碱，而大叶钩藤其嫩枝和叶的总碱含量平均为0.95%，因此过去对钩藤的挑选是不合理的，这个发现也解决了钩藤药材来源的紧张。

4. **各种生物碱都有不同的耐热性**　高温情况下某些生物碱不稳定，可产生水解、分解等变化。炮制常用煮、蒸、炒、烫、煅、炙等方法，改变生物碱的结构，以达到解毒、增效的目的。如士的宁在加热条件下转变为异士的宁、士的宁含氮氧化物等，保证临床用药安全。有些药物，如石榴皮、龙胆草、山豆根等所含的生物碱遇热活性降低，而所含生物碱又是有效物质，因而炮制过程中尽量减少热处理过程，以生用为宜。

Experiment 8　The Processing of Corydalis Rhizoma and Comparative Studies on the Alkaloids between the Crude and the Processed Drugs

Purpose

Compare the contenets of total alkoloids, in the water decoction between the crude Corydalis Rhizoma and the processed products, explain the changes of action and the meaning of the processing.

Principle

Rhizoma Corydlis is the dried tuber of *Corydalis yanhusuo* W. T. Wang. It can soothe the liver and regulate the flow of Qi, it also can promote the flow of Qi ande relieve the pain. According to the traditional Chinese medicine (TCM), it is used to relieve most kinds of pains widely.

According to the traditional Chinese medicine principle, vinegar can remove blood stasis and stop bleeding, and relieve pain. According to the TCM, processing with vinegar can increase. Corydalis's Rhizoma function about the soothing the liver ande relieving paining. Modern studies showed that Corydalis Rhizoma contains alkaloids mainly, have the obviusly function of relieving pain. After processed with vinegar, the amount of the total alkaloids and dl – tetrahydropalmatine (main effective component for relieving pain) increased in the water decoction. As a result, the effect of relieving pain will be increased.

dl-tetrahydropalmatine

Instruments and chemicals

1. Instruments

pot, spade, enamel plate, table balance, analytical balance, weighing bottle, baker, graduated cylinder, glass funnel, separate funnel, volumetric flask, vacum recovery apparatus, water bath, conical flask pipe, transfer pipet, basic buret (burette), electric oven.

2. Chemicals

Rice vinegar, ammonium hydroxide, chloroform, sodium slfate anhydrous, 0. 01mol/L sulfuric acid, 0. 02mol/L sodium hydroxide, methled – Bromocresol green indicater.

Experimental content

1. The processing of crude drugs

(1) Corydalis Rhizoma: Take crude Corydalis Rhizoma, to eliminae impurities and grey chip, wash clean dry and break into pieces.

(2) Cordalis Rhizoma stir – frying with vinegar: Mix up the clean Corydalis Rhizoma and rice vinegar. Cover tightly and moisten them until the rice vinegar is absorbed thoroughtly. Put Corydali Rhizoma in the pot and stir – fry with mild heating fire until the Corydalis Rhizoma dry. Take the drugs out from the pot. Chill before serving.

Every 100kg of Radix bupleuri, use 20kg of rice vinegar.

2. Determination of the total alkaloids

(1) The preparation of te samples: Take 10g of both the crude Corydalis Rhizoma and the processed Corydalis Rhizoma, weigh accurately, put them into two 500ml beakers respectively, then add 200ml, 100ml water to extract the drug for two times (Slightly boiling 20minutes for each time) respectively. Then filter the solution with cotton, mix the filtrate respectively. Add ammonium hydroxide to adjust pH value above 10, then transfer each filtrate to 250ml separating funnel.

To extract the filtrate with chloroform till the filtration showed negatve reaction with alkaloid reagents. Combine the extraction and wash with 20ml distilled water and then washed the water with 5ml chloroform. Combined the chloroform layer, add 5g sodium sulfate anhydrous to dehydration, and then to recovery the chloroform until the chloroform volume is very limited, then transfer the chloroform into 10 ml volumetric flask, add the chloroform to the scale.

(2) Assay ontotal alkaloids: Suck 5ml of above samples accurately, to 100ml conical flask. In ventilated kitchen, evaporate the chloroform on hot water bath, then add 2ml chloroform to dissolve the residue, add 20ml 0. 01mol/L sodium hydroxide. Add two drops of Methyl red and

Bromocresol green indicater. Titrate with 0.2mol/L sodium hydroxide. The end was indicated by the color changing from red into green). Calculate the content of total alkaloids (calculad by dl – tetrahydropalmatime).

$$Content(\%) = \frac{(N_{H_2SO_4} \cdot V_{H_2SO_4} - N_{NaOH} \cdot V_{NaOH}) \times 355.4}{W \times 1000} \times D \times 100\%$$

(D— dilutability)

Table 8 – 1   The content of total alkaloids

Samples	Weight(g)	Volume of NaOH (ml)	Content (%)
Crude Corydalis Rhizoma			
Processed Corydalis Rhizoma			

Experimental records

(1) Record content of total alkaloids experimental result, fill in the table 8 – 1.

(2) Make a record of the problems appeard during the experiment and explain the causes of the problems.

Matters needing attention

(1) The extraction by chloroform should be adequately, it is better according to "the smaller amount, the more times". If the emulsified layer appeared during the extraction by chloroform, we could use the glass rod stir it slightly to make the lay separate.

(2) The operation of evaporating the chloroform, should be in ventilated kitchen.

Reflection Questions

Compare the alkaloids amount between the crude drug and processed drug. What can you conclude according to the variation?

Related materials

The changes in traditional Chinese medicines containing alkaloid during the processing procedure.

Alkaloid is a kind of organic compounds containing nitrogen atoms. In general, alkaloids have a bitter taste. Many Chinese medicines, including herbs and animal medicines, contain some alkaloids. Because of these, we must pay attention to the changes of their physicochemical properties when we process drugs which contain alkaloids.

1. Free alkaloids in traditional Chinese medicines

Free alkaloids can be dissolved in organic solvents, so traditional Chinese medicinescontaining free alkaloids are usually processed with alcohol or yellow wine to increase the solubility of the alkaloids in water.

Free alkaloids can be dissolved in water when theycombine with some acids and become salts, so traditional Chinese medicines containing free alkaloids are usually processed with vinegar to increase the solubility of the alkaloids in water in order to increase their clinical effectiveness. For example, Corydalis Rhizomes (Yanhusuo) contains kinds of free alkaloid, and one of them, named Corybalis tetrahydropalmatine, is a very good analgesic. As a free alkaloid, it is less soluble in water. Some Research indicated that its solubility may be increased several times after Corydalis Rhizomes is stir – fried with vinegar. So the processed Rhizomes Corydalis has more effective in alleviating pain than the crude Corydalis Rhizomes.

2. Water – soluble alkaloid in traditional Chinese medicines

This kind of alkaloid is easy to be dissolved in water, such as arecaidine and berberine. For example, immerse traditional Chinese medicine into water for a long time when traditional Chinese medicines are softened, the water – soluble alkaloid can lose more from the Chinese medicines.

3. Alkaloids distributed in the different parts of a medicinal plant

Alkaloids are usually distributed in different parts of a medicinal plant. We can chose the some parts of plants in which there are more active components for the clinical application, and their clinical effectiveness was much better. For instance, Cortex Phellodendri (Huangbai) containing berberine (a main active alkaloid) was mainly made up of the cortical part of tree bark, expecially of its phloem. Therefore the cortex part was selected in the clinic of TCM, while the cork part was useless.

4. Toxic alkaloids in traditional Chinese medicines may be decreased

Alkaloid can be decomposed under the high temperature. According to this property, the toxic alkaloids can be turned into nontoxic or less toxic ones by boiling, steaming, stir – frying, and so on. For example, aconitine, is a toxic alkaloid of Radix Aconiti (Wutou) which have two ester bonds. Its toxicity is very strong. But aconitine can be broken up into aconine (which has lost two ester bonds from aconitine), which was less toxic, and whose effectiveness was kept.

实验九　炮制对黄连化学成分的影响

【实验目的】

1. 掌握黄连的炮制方法及原理。

2. 通过对黄连及其炮制品中生物碱含量的分析，从中选出最佳炮制工艺。

【实验原理】

黄连的主要成分为多种生物碱，主要有小檗碱、黄连碱、甲基黄连碱等。本实验原理，是以黄连中的有效成分小檗碱的含量为指标，利用溴麝香草酚蓝在 pH7.0 的水溶液中与小檗碱络合，形成 1∶1 的离子对的性质，再用三氯甲烷萃取，在 353nm 和 415nm 处测定吸收值，从而得到黄连中小檗碱的含量。另外，也可以利用小檗碱本身的结构特性——较长的共轭体系，在紫外区（349nm 处）有吸收，采用紫外分光度法进行测定。

小檗碱

【实验器材】

1. **仪器** 炒锅、锅铲、煤气灶、瓷盘（带盖）、切药刀、玻璃棒、研钵、9100 型分光光度计、离心机、分析天平（1/10000）、水浴锅、具塞离心管、索氏提取器、分液漏斗（60ml）、容量瓶（10ml，25ml）、微量注射器（50μl）、硅胶 G 薄层板（120℃活化）、吸量管（0.5ml、1ml、2ml、5ml）回收装置（圆底烧瓶、冷凝器、牛角导管、蒸馏头）、烧杯、玻璃漏斗、三角瓶、量筒。

2. **试剂** 正丁醇、冰醋酸、甲醇、乙醚、三氯甲烷、盐酸、溴麝香草酚蓝（均为AR.），蒸馏水、碘化铋钾（AR）、盐酸小檗碱标准品、黄连及其各炮制品粉末（过 60目筛）。

【实验内容】

一、黄连的炮制

1. **生黄连** 取原药材，拣去杂质，洗净泥沙，润透后切薄片，阴干，或用时捣碎。
2. **炒黄连** 将黄连片以文火炒至表面呈深黄色为度，取出放凉。
3. **酒黄连** 将黄连片置加盖容器内，加黄酒拌匀，闷润透（中间要搅拌数次），置热锅内，用文火炒至酒被吸干，取出放凉。

   每 100kg 黄连用黄酒 12.5kg。

4. **姜黄连** 将黄连片加姜汁拌匀，待吸收后，置炒锅内用文火炒至姜汁被吸尽，取出，放凉。

   每 100kg 黄连用生姜 12.5kg。

   鲜生姜汁制法：取鲜生姜，捣烂，榨汁，在加入药材中时，可兑入适量凉开水。

5. **吴萸连** 取吴茱萸加清水适量煎透，去药渣取煎液与黄连片拌匀，待吴茱萸被吸尽，用文火将黄连片炒干，取出晾干。

   每 100kg 黄连用吴茱萸 10kg。

二、黄连及其炮制品中小檗碱的测定

（一）方法一

1. **标准曲线的绘制** 精密称取盐酸小檗碱标准品 1.0mg，置 10ml 容量瓶中，加甲醇溶解稀释至刻度，制备成 0.1mg/ml 的标准溶液并精密量取 0.0ml、0.2ml、0.4ml、0.6ml、0.8ml、1.0ml，置 60ml 分液漏斗中，加溴麝香草酚蓝溶液 9ml 摇匀，精密加入三氯甲烷 10ml 振摇 1 分钟，放置待分层，分取三氯甲烷液，置干燥的具塞离心管中，

以每分钟 2500 转的速度，离心 2 分钟，置 1cm 石英吸收池中，在空白溶液的校正下，分别在 353nm 及 415nm 处测定吸收度，绘制标准曲线。

2. **小檗碱的测定**　取生黄连及其各种制品粉末（过 60 目筛）1.5g，置索氏提取器中，加入石油醚进行提取，1 小时后，倒出石油醚，换用甲醇回流提取至无色，回收甲醇，将提取液浓缩至 20ml 左右，将浓缩液转移至 25ml 容量瓶中，加蒸馏水至刻度，摇匀。用微量注射器吸取 50ml，在硅胶 G 薄层板上点样，以正丁醇∶冰醋酸∶水（7∶1∶2）为展开剂展开，挥去溶剂，在紫外灯下，刮取小檗碱的斑点，置索氏提取器中，用盐酸－甲醇（1∶100）洗脱，挥干溶剂，用量管取 3ml 蒸馏水，加入残渣中，置水浴中温热溶解残渣，放冷。精密量取 1ml，转移至分液漏斗中，加溴麝香草酚蓝溶液 9ml 摇匀，精密加入三氯甲烷 10ml 振摇 1 分钟，放置待分层，分取三氯甲烷液，置干燥的具塞离心管中，以每分钟 2500 转的速度，离心 2 分钟，置 1cm 石英吸收池中，在空白溶液的校正下，分别在 353nm 和 415nm 处测定吸光度（空白溶液为薄层板上空白硅胶 G 所得）。对照标准曲线，计算小檗碱含量。

$$小檗碱含量（\%）= \frac{C \times T}{W \times 1000} \times 100\%$$

式中，C 为由标准曲线查得的含量，mg；T 为稀释度；W 为饮片粉末重量。

（二）方法二

1. **标准曲线的制备**　精密称取盐酸小檗碱 0.075g，置 25ml 容量瓶中，加蒸馏水，在水浴上温热溶解，定容。吸取 0.00ml、0.25ml、0.50ml、1.00ml、1.50ml、2.00ml、2.50ml、3.00ml，分别置于 10ml 干燥容量瓶中，加入盐酸－甲醇（1∶100）溶液稀释至刻度，以盐酸甲醇溶液为空白对照，于 349nm 处测定吸收度，并绘制标准曲线。

2. **样品测定**　精密称取生黄连及黄连各炮制品粉末（过 60 目筛）1g，置索氏提取器中，加入甲醇 120ml，提取至无碘化铋钾反应，回收溶液，浓缩，定容于 10ml 容量瓶中，加盐酸－甲醇溶液稀释至刻度，以盐酸－甲醇溶液为空白对照，于 349nm 处测定吸收度，对照标准曲线，计算生物碱含量。

$$生物碱（\%）= \frac{C \times T}{W \times 1000} \times 100\%$$

式中，C 为由标准曲线得到的含量（mg）；T 为稀释度；W 为饮片粉末重量（g）。

表 9 - 1　小檗碱含量

样品	重量（g）	吸收度（A）	小檗碱含量（%）
生黄连			
炒黄连			
酒黄连			
姜黄连			
吴萸连			

【实验记录】

（1）记录黄连生、制品中小檗碱含量测定测定数据，填入表格。

（2）记录实验中出现的问题并说明原因。

【注意事项】

（1）炮制黄连时，注意火候，以免产生焦斑。

（2）测定生物碱含量时，要尽量保证生物碱提取完全。

【思考题】

（1）采用炒制、酒炙、姜炙、吴萸炙的黄连中的小檗碱含量有何不同，你认为该如何评价上述各种炮制方法？

（2）黄连中黄连素加热至220℃则转第为小檗红碱，从你的实验结果推测，有否这种转化，另外，黄连在炮制过程中有效成分流失的环节有哪些？

【相关资料】

黄连为毛茛科植物黄连 *Coptis chipensis* Franch. 三角叶黄连 *Coptis deltoidea* C. Y. Cheng et Hsiao. 或云连 *Coptis teeta* Wall 的根茎。以上三种分别习称"味连"、"雅连"、"云连"。秋季采挖，除去须根及泥沙，干燥，撞去残留须根。

黄连苦寒，入心、肝、胃、大肠经。有泻火、燥湿、解毒、杀虫之功。临床多用于湿热痞满，呕吐吞酸，泻痢，黄疸，高热神昏，心火亢盛，心烦不寐，血热吐衄，目赤，牙痛，消渴，痈肿疔疮；外治湿疹，湿疮，耳道流脓等。

Experiment 9　The Influence on Components of Coptidis Rhizoma by Processing

Purpose

1. To master the processing method and processing principle of Rhizoma coptidis.

2. To choice the best processing technology through analyzing the content of alkaloid in the Coptidis Rhizoma and its processed drug products.

Principle

Stir – frying Coptidis Rhizoma with wine or ginger can descend the nature of bitter cold of crude which processed with wine discharging fire from the upper part of the body. Stir – frying Coptidis Rhizoma with ginger can clean fire from the stomach, regulate the stomach function and relieve vomiting.

The main component of Coptidis Rhizoma are several kinds of alkaloids, such as berberine, coptisine, worenine, palmatine etc. .

The experiment study quality examination on all the processed Coptidis Rhizoma by the indicator of the content of active principle berberine in Coptidis Rhizoma. Method one: Using the character that berber complex with Bromothymol blue in pH 7.0 water liquid and become 1 : 1

ion pair. Then we extract the solution with trichloromethane and determine the absorbance at 353nm and 415nm. So we can calculate the berberine content in Coptidis Rhizoma. Method two: Berberine have absorption in ultraviolate region because of berberine's constitute character – fairly long conjugated system. In this experiment, determine the content of the berberine determined by means of Ultraviolet Sepctrophotometry.

berberine

Instruments and chemicals

1. Instruments

Pot, slice, gas cooker, porcelain dish (with cover), slicing knife, mortar, 9100 – type spectrophotometer, centrifuge, analytical balance (1/10000), water bath boiler, centrifuge tube (with cover), Soxhlet's extractor, separating funnel (60ml), volumetric flash (10ml, 25ml) microsyringe (50μl), silica gel G plate, measuring pipette (0.5ml, 1ml, 2, 5ml), recover unit (round flask, condensator, bubulum connecting conduct, distilling head), beaker, glass funnel, triangular flask, measuring cylinder.

2. Chemicals

n – butyl alcohol, hydrochloric acid, methanol, diethylether, chloroform, dilute potassium iodobismuthate (AR), distilled water, bromothymol blue (AR), good merchantable quality of hydrochloric acid berberine, the powder of Rhizoma Coptidis and its processed medicine (through a sieve of 60 items).

Experimental content

1. Processing

(1) Crude Coptidis Rhizoma: Take Coptidis Rhizoma, to eliminae impurities and grey chip, wash clean, cut into thin slices, dry it in air, or break to pieces before use.

(2) Stir – frying Coptidis Rhizoma: Stir – fry the slices with mild fire until the surface become deep yellow, then take out and cool.

(3) Stir – frying Coptidis Rhizoma with wine: Take the slices into the container (with cover), adding into rice wine, mix well. Then cover it until it is infused completely. Place the drugs in a pot and roast with slow fire to exhaust the wine. Take out and cool. 12.5kg Chinese rice wine is used for every 100kg Coptidis Rhizoma.

(4) Stir – frying Coptidis Rhizoma with ginger: Mix clean crude drugs with ginger – juice. Stir – fry in a pot with slow fire until the ginger – juice is absorbed completely. Take out and cool. Use 12.5kg ginger for each 100kg Coptidis Rhizoma.

Making fresh ginger – juice: Crush the fresh ginger to pasty, adding a quality of water, then get the juice.

(5) Stir – frying Coptidis Rhizoma with Fructus Evodiae: Decoct Fructus Evodiae with water. Add decoction to the clean Coptidis Rhizoma until decoction is absorbed completely. Use Fructus Ebodiae 10kg for each 100kg Coptidis Rhizoma.

2. Determination of berberine

Method 1

(1) Draw the calibration curve: Take about 1.0mg of good merchantable quality of hydrochloric acid berberine weigh accurately. Put it into 10ml volumetric flask, dilute with methanol to volume and the solution containing 0.1mg hydrochloric acid berberine per ml. Measure accurately 0.0, 0.2, 0.4, 0.6, 0.8 and 1.0ml, respectively, into 60ml separating funnel. Add 9ml bromothymol blue, and mix well. Measure accurately 10ml chloroform into it, shaking out for 1 minute, standing still the solution separate, getting the chloroform to centrifuge tube (with cover), centrifuge for 2 minutes at the speed of 2500 per minute. Determine the absorbance at 353nm and 415nm respectively. Make calibration curve.

(2) Dertermination of berberine: Take 1.5g of powder of crude and every kind of processed Rhizoma Coptidis to Soxhlet's extractor. Add light petroleum and extract for 1 hour, eliminate light petroleum. Add methanol and extract until the extract is colorless. Remove methanol. Concentrate the solution to 20ml. Put the concentrate to 25ml volumetric flask, dilute with distilled water to volume, and mix well. Measure accurately 50μl by microsyringe, and then inject it on the silica gel G, developing by n – butylalcohol : hydrochloric acid: water(7:1:2). Take the spot of fluorescent into Soxhelt's extracrtor. Add hydrochloric acid – methanol (1:100) and volatilize until no solution. Add 3ml of distilled water to residual and dissolve it in water bath. After cooling take accurately 1ml into funnel. Add 9ml bromothymol blue, and mix well. Measure accurately 10ml chloroform into it, shaking out for 1 minute, standing still the solution separate, getting the chloroform to centrifuge tube (with cover), centrifuge for 2 minutes at the speed of 2500 per minute. Determine the absorbance at 353nm and 415nm respectively. Calculate the content of berberine comparing calibration curve.

$$\text{Berberine}(\%) = \frac{C \times T}{W \times 1000} \times 100\%$$

C—content from calibration curve, mg

T—dilution

W—weight of drug powder, g

Method 2

(1) Drawing of the calibration curve: Take about 0.075g of standard substance of hydrochloric acid berberine weigh accurately. Put it into 25ml volumetric flask. Put into distilled water and dissolve it to volume in water bath. Measure accurately 0.00, 0.25, 0.50, 1.00, 1.50, 2.00, 2.50 and 3.00ml and put them separately into 10ml volumetric flask. Add hydro-

chloric acid – methanol (1:100) to volume. Determine the absorance at 349nm. Make calibration curve.

(2) Determination of alkaloids: Take 1g of powder of crude and every kind of processed Coptidis Rhizoma, weigh accurately. Put it into Soxhlet's extractor. Add 120ml of methanol and extract until no bismuth potassium iodide reaction, remove methanol. Dissolve the concentrate solution with hydrochloric acid – methanol and take it to 10ml volumetric flask. Dilute with hydrochloric acid – methanol to volume. Determine the absorbance at 349nm. Calculate the content of alkaloid comparing calibration curve.

$$Alkaloid(\%) = \frac{C \times T}{W \times 1000} \times 100\%$$

C—content from calibration curve, mg

T—dilution

W—weight of drug powder, g

Table 9 – 1　Content of berberine

Samples	Weight(g)	Absorbance(A)	Content of berberine(%)
Crude Coptidis Rhizoma			
Stir – frying Coptidis Rhizoma			
Stir – frying with wine			
Stir – frying with ginger			
Stir – frying with Fructus Evodiae			

Experimental records

(1) Record every experimental data of determine of total alkaloids and berberine, fill in the table 9 – 1.

(2) Make a record of the problems appeard during the experiment and explain the causes of the problems.

Matters needing attention

(1) Pay attention to the optimal fire as processing for fear that produce burnt spot.

(2) To sure all the alkaloid is extracted absolutely in the experiment which the content of alkaloid was determined.

Reflection Questions

(1) What the difference of the content of berberine in each processed Rhizoma Coptidis?

(2) Researches showed that berberine invests into berberubine when it was heated to 220℃. Do you have the same deduction from your experiment result?

Related materials

Huanglian is the dried rhizome of *Coptis chinensis* Franch, *Coptis deltoidea* C. Y. Cheng et Hsiao, *Coptis omeiensis* (Chen) C. Y. Cheng and *Coptis teetoides* C. Y. Cheng.

The source of Coptidis Rhizoma is from Rhizome of *Coptis chinensis* Franch. and C. deltoidea C. Y. Cheng et Hsiao or *Coptis teetoides* C. Y. Cheng, family Ranunculaceae. The producing areas are mainly in the provinces of Sichuan and Yunnan. The medicinal material is dug and collected in autumn and dried.

Coptidis Rhizoma is bitter in flavor, cold in nature and attributive to the heart, liver, stomach and large intestine meridians. It is used for dysentery and vomiting of dampness – heat type. It has a strong action of clearing away heat and eliminating dampness and is especially good at removing heat and dampness from the middle energizer, and serves as an essential medicinal herb for treatment of diarrhea and dysentery of damp – heat type. Coptidis Rhizoma can be used to cure directly epidemic heat toxins, typhoid, excessive heat and vexation, retching and hiccup due to feeling of fullness in the bosom and upper abdomen, toothache due to stomach – fire, vomiting due to stomach – heat, pulmonary tuberculois, vomit the blood, diabetes, infantile malnutrition, ascariasis, swollen sore throat, fire – eyes, aphthae, suppurative skin diseases, infantile eczema, scald etc. .

实验十 煅 法

【实验目的】

1. 掌握明煅法、煅淬法和闷煅法的操作技术及成品质量要求。
2. 了解煅法的目的和意义。

【实验原理】

将药物直接置于无烟炉火中或置于适宜的耐火容器内煅烧的一种方法称为煅法。煅法可分为明煅法、煅淬法和闷煅法3种，主要适用于矿物类、动物贝壳类及质地轻松而煅炭的药物。药物经煅制后，可使其质地酥脆，有利于粉碎和有效成分的煎出，亦可减少或消除毒副作用。

明矾为天然矾石或其他铝矿石经加工提炼制成的硫酸钾铝结晶，具有收敛止血、收湿止痒作用。经煅制后，其收敛燥湿作用增强。其炮制原理为：

$$KAl(SO_4)_2 \cdot 12H_2O \rightarrow KAl(SO_4)_2 + 12H_2O$$

血余炭是人发经闷煅制成的炭化物，具有止血作用，本品不生用，煅炭后使其 Ca^{2+} 和 Fe^{2+} 易于煎出。

【实验器材】

炉子、铁铲、锅、坩埚、烧杯、量筒、火钳、电炉、大小瓷蒸发皿、搪瓷盘、台秤、马福炉、盐泥、米醋等。

【实验内容】

一、明煅法

1. **明矾** 取明矾，除去杂质，筛或拭去浮灰，打碎，称重，置于适宜的容器内，用武火加热，切勿搅拌，煅至水分完全蒸发，无气体放出，全部松泡，呈白色蜂窝状固体时，取出放凉，称重。

成品性状：本品呈洁白色，无光泽，蜂窝状块，体轻松，手捻易碎。

2. 石膏 取净石膏块，称重，置适宜容器内或直接置火源上，用武火加热，煅至红透，取出放凉，碾细，称重。

成品性状：本品煅后呈洁白色或粉条状或块状，表面松脆，易剥落，光泽消失，手捻易碎。

3. 龙骨 取净龙骨，敲成小块，称重，置适宜容器内，用武火加热，煅至红透，取出放凉，称重。

成品性状：本品呈灰白色或灰褐色，质酥脆，吸舌力强。

二、煅淬法

1. 自然铜 取净自然铜小块，置适宜容器内，用武火加热，煅至红透，取出后立即放入醋内浸淬，如此反复煅淬数次，至黑褐色，表面光泽消失并酥松，取出，摊晾。

每100kg 自然铜，用米醋30kg。

成品性状：本品为不规则碎粒，灰黑色或黑褐色，质酥脆，无金属光泽。带醋气。

2. 代赭石 取净代赭石碎块，置适宜容器内或直接置火源上，用武火加热，煅至红透，取出后立即放入醋内浸淬，如此反复煅淬数次，直至酥脆，取出干燥，碾成细粉。

每100kg 代赭石，用米醋30kg。

成品性状：本品呈暗褐色或紫褐色，光泽消失，略带醋气。

三、扣锅煅法（密闭煅法）

1. 灯心草 取净灯心草，扎成小把，置适宜容器内，上扣一较小容器，两容器结合处用盐泥封固，上压重物，并贴一块白纸条或放大米数粒，先用文火加热，后用武火煅至白纸或大米呈深黄色时，停火，待凉后，取出。

成品性状：呈炭黑色，有光泽。质轻松，易碎。

2. 血余炭 取头发除去杂质，反复用稀碱水洗去油垢，清水漂净，晒干，置适宜容器内，上扣一较小容器，两容器结合处用盐泥封固，上压重物，并贴一块白纸条或放大米数粒，先用文火加热，后用武火煅至白纸或大米呈深黄色时，停火，待凉后，取出。

成品性状：本品为不规则的小块状，乌黑光亮，呈蜂窝状，研之清脆有声，质轻易碎，有不快的臭气。

【**实验记录**】

（1）记录明煅法、煅淬法和闷煅法中各种药物形态、颜色、气味的变化。

（2）记录实验中出现的问题并说明原因。

【**注意事项**】

（1）在明矾煅制过程中，不能停火，亦不能搅拌，应一次煅透，使其完全失去结晶水。

（2）明矾的煅制最佳温度为 180℃ ~ 260 ℃，不得超过 600℃，否则 KAl（SO₄）₂分解，损失药效。

（3）煅锅内药物不宜放得过多、过紧，以容器的 2/3 为宜。

（4）血余炭闷煅时，应防止漏气，免使药物灰化；且以滴水于盖锅的四周即沸或盖锅上四周的白纸呈焦黄色为宜。煅制后，不可立即开锅，应充分冷却后打开锅。

【思考题】

（1）实验中各药炮制目的是什么？

（2）煅制三法各有何特点？分别适用于哪类药材？

Experiment 10 Calcined Method

Purpose

1. To master the processing method of calcining method, including direct calcining method, calcined quenching method and airtight calcined method.

2. To understand the processing purpose of calcining method.

Principle

Calcining is a kind of method treating crude medicinal materials by direct or indirect burning with medium heating or strong fire. Calcining contain 3 kind of method including direct calcining method, calcined quenching method, and airtight calcined method.

The purposes are to make them pure, clean, crispy, easy to be powdered and their effective components decocted out or their natures change to produce better therapeutic effects. Some crude medicinal herbs of hard minerals or shells may be burned directly till they are thoroughly reddish, then they are quickly put into vinegar or clean water, which is called tempering.

The processing principle of White Alum can be explained as:

$$KAl(SO_4)_2 \cdot 12H_2O \rightarrow KAl(SO_4)_2 + 12H_2O$$

Instruments

Pot, stove, shovel, ceramic bowl, sieve, thermometer, balance, parallel avertense.

Experimental Contents

1. Direct calcining method

（1）White alum (Mingfan): Dried alum: Take the clean alum. Break into small lumps. Place into the pan and calcine with strong fire to be melting and go on to make them expanded like honeycomb. Stop heating while it is dried thoroughly. Take the drugs out from the pot and cool it.

（2）Gypsum Fibrosum (Shigao): Calcined gypsum Fibrosum : Take the clean calcined gypsum Fibrosum. Break into small lumps. Place into the fireproof container. Calcine it with strong fire until it is red thoroughly. Take the drugs out and cool it. Grind it.

（3）Ossa draconis（Longgu）：Calcined Ossa draconis：Take the clean Ossa draconis. Break into small lumps. Place into the fireproof container. Calcine it with strong fire until it is red thoroughly. Take the drugs out and cool it. Grind it.

2. Calcined quenching method

（1）Pyritum（Zirantong）：Calcined pyritum：Take the clean pyritum. Break into small lumps. Place into the fireproof container. Calcine it with strong fire until it is red thoroughly. Dip it into the vinegar immediately for quenching. Take the drugs out from the vinegar. Go on to calcine and quench until it is blackish brown without metalluster, and crisp in texture. Take it out. Grind it after it is dried.

Use 30kg vinegar for every 100kg pyritum.

（2）Red Ochre（Daizheshi）：Calcined red ochre：Take the clean red ochre. Break into small lumps. Place into the fireproof container. Calcine it with strong fire until it is red thoroughly. Dip it into the vinegar immediately for quenching. Take the drugs out from the vinegar. Go on to calcine and quench until it is crisp in texture. Take it out. Grind it after it is dried.

Use 30kg vinegar every 100kg red ochre.

3. Airtight calcined method

（1）Junci Medulla（Dengxincao）：Charred Junci Medulla：Take clean Junci Medulla into the altithermal endurably crucible, leave certain place when putting the drugs into the crucible, cover a smaller caliber pot, seal the junction with salt mud or sand buckle on container, two container junction with salt mud or fine sand. Press with some heavy, dip a piece of paper or place a few grains of rice on the bottom of the upper pot as the mark. Heat it with strong fire until the paper or rice appears dark yellow. Stop heating. Take it out when it is cool enough.

（2）Crinis Carbonisatus（Xueyutan）：Charred crinis carbonisatus：Take the hair. Get rid of the impurities. Wash with dilute basic water repeatedly. Rinse with clean water. Dry it in the sun. Put them in the pot, leave certain place when putting the drugs into the crucible, cover a smaller caliber pot, seal the junction with salt mud or sand buckle on container, two container junction with salt mud or fine sand. Press with some heavy, dip a piece of paper or place a few grains of rice on the bottom of the upper pot as the mark. Heat it with strong fire until the paper or rice appears dark yellow. Stop heating. Take it out when it is cold enough.

Experimental records

（1）Record the changes of form, color and odour during the processing of direct calcining method, calcined quenching method and airtight calcined method.

（2）Make a record of the problems appeard during the experiment and explain the causes of the problems.

Matters needing attention

（1）In alum calcined process, not a cease – fire, nor stir, shall be a burnt, make its crystallization water completely lost.

（2）The temperature of the alum calcined temperature is 180 ℃ ～ 260 ℃, shall not exceed

600 ℃ ,otherwise ,the effect will reduce.

（3）Burnt pot drugs should not be too much ,and not be too tight ,With two – thirds of container advisable.

（4）Carbonized human hair stuffy calcined ,should prevent gas leakage ,free drug ashing. Open the pot after fully cooled.

Questions

（1）What is the main processing purpose of these drugs?

（2）What is the character of three kinds of calcining methods? Which crude drug is fit for these three kinds of calcining methods ,respectively?

实验十一　蒸法及不同软化方法对黄芩中黄芩苷的影响

【实验目的】

1. 掌握蒸法的基本操作方法。

2. 掌握黄芩最佳软化方法。

3. 通过不同软化方法的比较，说明黄芩蒸法软化的意义。

【实验原理】

现代研究表明，黄芩遇冷水变绿，就是由于黄芩中所含的酶在一定温度和湿度条件下，可酶解黄芩中所含的黄芩苷和汉黄芩苷，产生葡萄糖醛酸和两种苷元，即黄芩素和汉黄芩素。其中黄芩苷元是一种邻位三羟基黄酮，本身不稳定，容易被氧化而变绿。故黄芩变绿说明黄芩苷已被水解。黄芩苷的水解又与酶的活性有关，以冷水浸，酶的活性最大。而"蒸"和"煮"或炒制就可以破坏酶，使其活性消失，有利于黄芩苷的保存。黄芩蒸制或沸水煮的目的是使酶灭活，保存药效，又能使药物软化，便于切片。

黄芩苷

黄芩酶

黄色　→　[O]　→　绿色

【实验器材】

1. 仪器　蒸锅、小三角瓶、具塞三角烧瓶、天平、滤纸、毛细管、层析缸、薄层层析板。

2. 试剂　黄芩苷、硅胶 G、0.5% CMC – Na 溶液、甲苯、甲酸、乙酸乙酯、乙醇。

【实验内容】

1. 地黄、大黄的蒸制

（1）地黄的蒸制　取净生地黄，置蒸制容器内，隔水蒸至黑润，取出，晒至八成干，切厚片，干燥。

（2）大黄的蒸制　取大黄片或块，用黄酒拌匀，闷润至酒被吸尽，装入蒸制或炖制容器内，密闭，隔水炖至大黄内外均呈黑色时，取出，干燥。

每 100kg 大黄片或块，用黄酒 30kg。

2. 黄芩药材的软化、切片

（1）冷浸软化切片　取原药材，除去杂质，洗净。加 10 倍量冷水，冷浸 12 小时，取出，切薄片。干燥。

（2）蒸法软化切片　取原药材，除去杂质，洗净。大小分档，置蒸制容器内隔水加热，蒸至"圆汽"后半小时，候质地软化，取出，趁热切薄片。干燥。

3. 定性实验

（1）制硅胶 G 板　取硅胶 G 适量，加入 2.5 ~ 2.7 倍的 0.5% CMC – Na 溶液搅匀，适当研磨，倒在玻璃上，待自然干燥后放入烘箱，于 110℃ 活化半小时，取出后放入干燥器中备用。

（2）样品的制备　取干燥的生品（冷浸软化切片）及蒸制黄芩片（蒸法软化切片）分别粉碎，各取 0.2g 置小三角瓶中，加蒸馏水 2ml，放置 24 小时，观察记录色泽变化，然后各加 95% 乙醇 8ml，立即放入 80℃ 水浴中加热 10 分钟，分别滤于小三角烧瓶中，供点样用。

（3）点样及展开　取上述制备的样品液及黄芩苷、黄芩苷元对照品，用毛细管点于薄层板上，置于层析槽内，以甲苯 – 乙酸乙酯 – 甲酸（3:3:1）为展开剂展开，挥干溶剂，观察结果并计算其 R_f 值。

【实验记录】

（1）记录薄层层析结果，拍照并画图，对结果进行解释。

（2）记录薄层层析中出现的问题并说明原因。

【注意事项】

实验操作时，样品和对照品力求条件一致，否则影响结果。

【思考题】

（1）如何确定黄芩切片前软化的最佳方法？

（2）从哪些指标可以评价黄芩饮片的质量？

【相关资料】

1. 黄芩　为唇形科植物黄芩 *Scutellaria baicalensis* Geogi 的干燥根。主产于东北、河北、山西，内蒙古等地。春、秋两季采挖，除去须根及泥沙，晒后撞去粗皮，晒干。

黄芩味苦，性寒。归肺、胆、脾、大肠、小肠经。具有清热燥湿、泻火解毒、止血、安胎的功能。

2. 炮制对含苷类药物的影响 苷系糖分子中环状半缩醛上的羟基与非糖部分（苷元）中的羟基（或酚基）缩合（失水）而成的环状缩醛衍生物。苷溶解性能无明显规律，一般易溶于水或乙醇中。苷键是苷分子特有的化学键，它有糖的端基碳上形成的缩醛结构，具有一般缩醛的性质，如对酸不稳定性。苷键裂解的方式有酸催化水解、碱催化水解、酶催化水解、氧化开裂反应等。炮制过程中苷键的断裂一般有这些反应的参与。

由于苷类成分易溶于水，所以中药在炮制过程中用水处理时尽量少泡多润，以免苷类物质溶于水而流失或发生水解而减少。常见者如大黄、甘草、秦皮等，均含可溶于水的各种苷，切制用水处理时要特别注意。

不同的炮制方法可直接影响其含量。含苷类成分的中药往往在不同细胞中含有相应的酶，这种酶能使其共存的苷在一定的温度和湿度条件下分解，从而使有效成分减少，影响疗效。如黄芩、苦杏仁等含苷中药，采收后长期放置，相应的酶便可分解黄芩苷、苦杏仁苷，从而使这些中药失效。如黄芩苷的水解与酶的活性有关，以冷水浸活性最大，而蒸或煮可破坏酶使其活性消失，有利于黄芩苷的保存。现代研究表明，黄芩遇冷水变绿，就是由于黄芩中所含的酶在一定的温度和湿度下，可酶解黄芩中所含的黄芩苷产生黄芩苷元，是一种邻位三羟基黄酮，本身不稳定，容易被氧化而变绿。故黄芩变绿说明黄芩苷已被水解。黄芩苷的水解又与酶的活性有关，以冷水浸，酶的活性最大。而黄芩蒸制就可破坏酶，使其活性消失，有利于黄芩苷的保存。

与此类似，苦杏仁、芥子等中药，同样含有苷和酶类，通常采用蒸、炒制等加热的方法处理，中药炮制中称为"杀酶保苷"。

苷类成分的另一个特点是在酸性条件下容易水解，不但减低了苷的含量，也增加了成分的复杂性，因此，炮制时除医疗上有专门要求外，一般少用或不用醋处理。在生产过程中，有机酸会被水或醇溶出，使水呈酸性，促进苷的水解，应加以注意。但某些药物，可以通过醋炙降低毒性，例如商陆，含有毒性苷类成分，醋炙后含量降低，毒性降低，所以中医临床上主要使用醋商陆。

Experiment 11   The Processing Method of Steaming and Effect of Different Softing Methods to Baicalin in Radix Scutellariae and the Assay by means of TLC

Purpose

1. To master the processing method of steaming.

2. To master the best softening method of Radix Scutellariae.

3. To study the principle and significance of processing through the comparison of the ba-

icalin content after and before processing.

Principle

Modern study showed thatthe main active constituent of Radix Scutellariae (Huangqin) is baicaline which having yellow color can be broken down into Baicalein by enzyme in the herbs. The baicalein is not stable and easy to be oxygenated into a kind of quinones which color is green. As a result that Radix Scutellariae will change green in cold water due to the oxidization of the baicalin. Since the hydrolysis of baicalin depend on the activity of the enzyme, and Radix Scutellariae soaked in cold water possessing, thestrong activity of enzyme will lead massive baicalin to lose. While the drugs processed through steaming, boiling or stir – frying can reserve most baicalin because the heat processing can destroy the enzyme to protect the baicalin, meanwhile, steaming can softening drugs to the benefit of cutting slice.

The baicalin can be determined throughTLC, and used to evaluate the quality of drugs. Through the changing of effective component, we can study the principle and significance of Radix Scutellariae processing.

Instruments and chemicals

1. Instruments

Steaming pot, small triangle bottle, triangle bottle with a plug, balance, filter paper, capillary tubesaturate tank, glassplate.

2. Chemtcals

Baicalin, CMC – Na solution, methylbenzene, formic acid, ethyl acetate, ethyl alcohol, yellow rice or millet wine.

Experimental content

1. The processing method of steaming Radix Rehmanniae and Radix et Rhizoma Rhei

(1) Radix Rehmanniae: Eliminate foreign matter, steamRadix Rehmanniae until it becomes blackish and shiny, take out, dry in the sun to be eighty percent dried, then cut into

thick slices and dry.

(2) Radix et Rhizoma Rhei: Eliminate foreign matter, stirRadix et Rhizoma Rhei with yellow rice or millet wine. Cover tightly and moisten them until the yellow rice or millet wine is absorbed thoroughtly. Put it into airtight container, stew it until the interior and exterior of the drugs become black. Take out, dry it.

Every 100kg ofRadix et Rhizoma Rhei, use 30 kg ofyellow rice or millet wine.

2. The softening and section of drugs.

(1) Radix Scutellariae immersed in cold water: Immersed the raw drugs (200g) with 2000ml water for 12h, removed and cool to dry.

(2) Radix Scutellariae steamed with hot water: Eliminate foreign matter, steam for half an hour, take out, then cut into thin slices and dry, protecting from exposure to strong sunlight.

3. Comparison on different processed products of Fructus Aurantii by TLC method.

(1) Preparation of Silica gel G plate: Take Silica gel Gmoderately, adding 2.5 ~ 2.7 times 0.5% CMC – Na solution, mix up, grinding. Pour it on the glassplate, dry it. At 110℃ activation about a half hours. Take it out, put it in the dryer, standby application.

(2) Sample preparation: Take the crude drug andsteamed product of Fructus Aurantii 0.2ginto small triangle bottlerespectively. Add 2ml distilled water, place it about 24 hours. Observe and record the change of colour and luster. Add 95% ethyl alcohol 8ml, put it in80℃ water bath, heat it 10minutes, filter into thesmall triangle flask, respectively, standby application.

(3) Sample points and spread in TLC: Take equivalent crude drug and processed product of Fructus Aurantii solution, and baicalin, baicalin, point on the same silica G thin layer plate respectively. Use methylbenzene – ethyl acetate – methanoic acid (3:3:1), as developing solvent. Take out to dry. Discuss the influence of the chemical composition because of processing according to the number, size and colorof spots. Calculate the Rf value.

Experimental records

1. Record the TLC result, take pictures and draw it. Explain the results.

2. Make a record of the problems appeard during in the TLC experiment and illustrate the causes of the problems.

Matters needing attention

During the experimental operation, the condition sample should be consistent, otherwise it will influence the experimental results.

Reflection Questions

1. How to determine the best method to process radix scutellariae before cutting?

2. Which indicator can be used for assessment of radix scutellariaeslices?

Related materials

1. Radix Scutellariae (Huangqin)

The source is from the root of *Scutellaria baicalensis* Georgi, family Labiatae. It is mainly produced in the provinces of Hebei, Shanxi and inner Mongolia autonomous region, etc. , digged up and collected in spring and autumn, usually cut into pieces, the crude one and the one stir – baked with wine or the carbonized one may be used.

It can be used in such indications as discomfort in test, nausea and vomiting in epidemic febrile diseases caused by damp – heat or summer – heat; cough due to heat in the lung; high fever with fire thirst; spitting of blood and epistaxis due to heat in blood ; carbuncles and sores; threatened avortion. The crude drug is good at removing damp – heat. While the processed products (processing with wine) is especially good for the diseases of eye sore, heat in lung and the damp – heat in limb and skin because the wine can lead it into the blood and aid the ascending power. After processed with wine (with the heat property of wine) , the cold property of the drugs is decreased, so as to avoid injuring the spleen and stomach.

2. The changes of glycosides in Chinese herbs during the processing procedures.

Glycoside exists in the Chinese herbs widely, and it is easy to be dissolved in water and alcohol. The method of softening the drugs which contain glycosides must be taken seriously.

In general, there are glycosides and enzymes hydrolyzing them in the same medicinal herbs. The enzyme can hydrolyze the glycoside into aglycone under certain temperature and moisture. This hydrolyzing reaction can occur in the interior of medicinal herbs at ordinary condition. This will lead the active glycosides of these drugs changed and their effect reduced.

For example, the main active constituent of Radix Scutellariae (Huangqin) is baicaline which having yellow color can be broken down into baicalein by enzyme in the herbs. The baicalein is not stable and easy to be oxygenated into a kind of quinones which color is green. The processing principle of this medicine has been revealed, that is the yellow Radix Scutellariae is better than the green one on the therapeutic effectiveness. So the steaming method for softening Radix Scutellariae has been used universally acknowledged in China.

Semen Armeniacae amarum (Kuxingren) is processed by steaming or stir – frying, SemenSinapis (Jiezi) is processed by stir – frying, so the enzymes are destroyed at the higher temperatures and the glycosides are kept. That is the means of a professional term "Killing enzymes and protecting glycosides" .

Another property of glycosides is that they can be decomposed in the acidic conditions. Therefore, most of herbs containing glycosides aren't processed with vinegar. But a few of drugs are processed with vinegar to reduce their toxicity. For example, Radix Phytolaccae (Shanglu) contains phytolaccoside – B as a bio – active component haing strong toxicity. The toxicity of processed product with vinegar is weaker than the crude drug. So Radix Phytolaccae processed product with vinegar was used in clinic of TCM.

实验十二　煮法及乌头煮制前后生物碱的含量及毒性变化

【实验目的】

1. 掌握煮法的基本炮制方法。

2. 通过炮制前后乌头中所含生物碱的含量及毒性变化，说明药材炮制的目的和意义。

【实验原理】

煮法可以降低乌头等药物的毒副作用，并可增强药效，改变药性。

乌头分川乌、草乌两种，生品均有大毒，多做外用，煮制后毒性降低，可供内服。乌头的毒性成分主要为双酯型生物碱，煮制或蒸制后双酯型生物碱被水解形成单酯型生物碱，其毒性为双酯型乌头碱的 1/500 ~ 1/200，进一步水解形成乌头原碱，其毒性仅为双酯型乌头碱的 1/4000 ~ 1/2000，从而降低毒性。

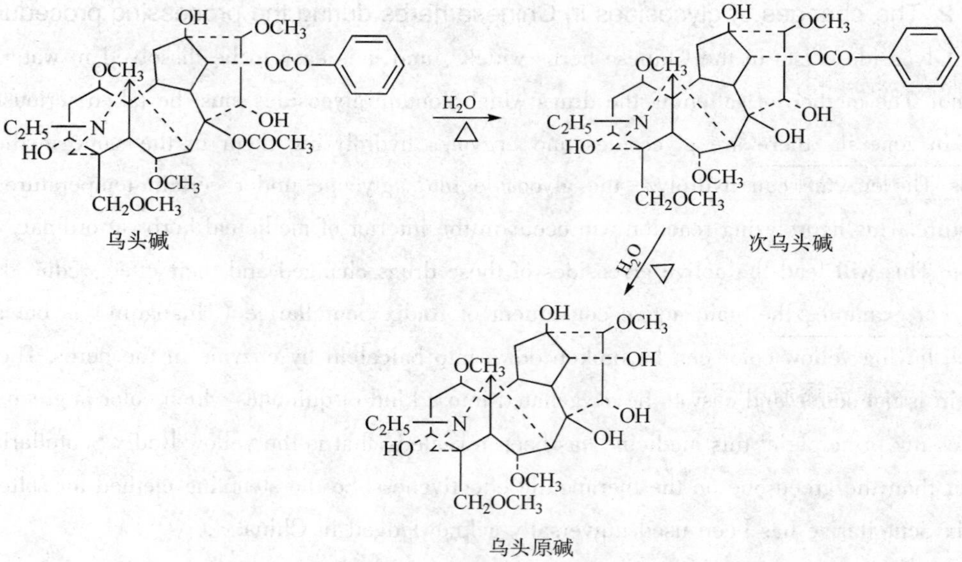

图 12 – 1　乌头碱水解反应

【实验器材】

1. **仪器**　蒸锅、高压锅、天平、漏斗、高效液相色谱仪、超声波清洗器、微量进样器、微孔滤膜、50ml 具塞锥形瓶、50ml 移液管、5ml 移液管。

2. **试剂**　苯甲酰乌头原碱标准品、苯甲酰次乌头原碱标准品、苯甲酰新乌头原碱标准品、乌头碱标准品、次乌头碱标准品、新乌头碱标准品、氨试液、乙腈（色谱纯）、四氢呋喃（色谱纯）、0.1mol/L 醋酸铵溶液、冰醋酸、异丙醇（色谱纯）、三氯甲烷（色谱纯）、乙酸乙酯。

【实验内容】

一、煮法

1. 乌头的炮制 取生乌头100g，洗去泥沙，大小分档，水浸泡至内无干心，取出，置蒸锅内，加水（浸泡过乌头表面）煮沸4~6小时，或蒸制6~8小时，也可放入高压锅煮50分钟左右，至切开内无白心，口尝微有麻舌感，取出切薄片，晒干或烘干（80℃以下约3小时）。

2. 成品性状 表面黑褐色，质脆，气微，微有麻舌感。

3. 炮制作用 生乌头有大毒，多外用。炮制后降低乌头毒性，可供内服。

二、生物碱的含量测定

高效液相色谱法

1. 色谱条件与系统适用性试验 以十八烷基硅烷键合硅胶为填充剂，以乙腈－四氢呋喃（25:15）为流动相A，以0.1mol/L醋酸铵溶液（每1000ml加冰醋酸0.5ml）为流动相B，按表12－1中的规定进行梯度洗脱；检测波长为235nm。理论板数按苯甲酰新乌头原碱峰计算应不低于2000。

表12－1 梯度洗脱程序

时间（分钟）	流动相A（%）	流动相B（%）
0~48	15→26	85→74
48~48.1	26→35	74→65
48.1~58	35	65
58~65	35→15	65→85

2. 对照品溶液的制备 取苯甲酰乌头原碱对照品、苯甲酰次乌头原碱对照品、苯甲酰新乌头原碱对照品适量，精密称定，加异丙醇－三氯甲烷（1:1）混合溶液分别制成每1ml含苯甲酰乌头原碱20μg、苯甲酰次乌头原碱0.1mg、苯甲酰新乌头原碱80μg的混合溶液，即得。

3. 供试品溶液的制备 取生、制乌头粉末（过三号筛）约2g，精密称定，置具塞锥形瓶中，加氨试液3ml，精密加入异丙醇－乙酸乙酯（1:1）混合溶液50ml，称定重量，超声处理（功率300W，频率40kHz；水温在25℃以下）30分钟，放冷，再称定重量，用异丙醇－乙酸乙酯（1:1）混合溶液补足减失的重量，摇匀，滤过。精密量取续滤液25ml，40℃以下减压回收溶剂至干，残渣精密加入异丙醇－三氯甲烷（1:1）混合溶液3ml溶解，滤过，取续滤液，即得。

测定法：分别精密吸取对照品溶液与供试品溶液各10μl，注入液相色谱仪，测定，即得。

双酯型生物碱照上述色谱条件和供试品溶液的制备方法试验。

4. 对照品溶液的制备 取乌头碱对照品、次乌头碱对照品及新乌头碱对照品适量，精密称定，加异丙醇－三氯甲烷（1:1）混合溶液分别制成每1ml含乌头碱30μg、次乌头碱10μg、新乌头碱50μg的溶液，即得。

测定法：分别精密吸取对照品溶液与供试品溶液各10μl，注入液相色谱仪，测定，即得。

三、炮制前后乌头的毒性实验

1. **样品试液的制备**　取生、制乌头粉各20g，分别加入蒸馏水200ml，加热煮制30分钟，滤过，残渣再加蒸馏水煮两次，滤过，合并滤液，浓缩至10%供试品溶液，滤过。

2. **毒性实验**　取体重18～22g的小白鼠40只，随机分成2组，分别标号称重，然后腹腔注射生、制乌头供试品溶液（0.5ml/10g）。观察2小时，记录动物中毒症状、死亡时间和死亡数。

【实验记录】

（1）记录生物碱的含量测定、毒性实验的实验结果。

（2）记录实验中出现的问题并说明原因。

【注意事项】

乌头有大毒，操作时注意安全。

【思考题】

（1）乌头有哪些炮制方法，这些炮制方法有什么异同点？

（2）乌头炮制的作用及作用原理怎样？

Experiment 12　The Method of Boiling and its Influence on the Content and Toxicity of Alkaloid in Aconite Root

Purpose

1. To master the method of boiling.

2. To illustrate the purpose and signification of processing by comparing the content and toxicity of alkaloid in the raw and the processed drugs.

Principle

Boiling method can remove or decrease the drug's toxicity, alter drug's property and strengthen the therapeutic effectiveness.

Aconite root include Aconiti Radix and Aconiti Kusnezoffii Radix, which are both hyper-toxic, and mostly used externally, boiling can reduce the toxicity of the drug and can be used orally. The toxic constituent of aconite root is alkaloid which posses double ester bonds, and can be hydrolyzed to single ester bond alkaloid by boiling or steaming, which toxicity is 1/500—1/200 of that of diester type. Single ester bond alkaloid can be hydrolyzed to alkaloid by further boiling or steaming to produce aconine, which toxicity is 1/4000—1/2000 of that of diester type alkaloid to decrease the toxicity of drug.

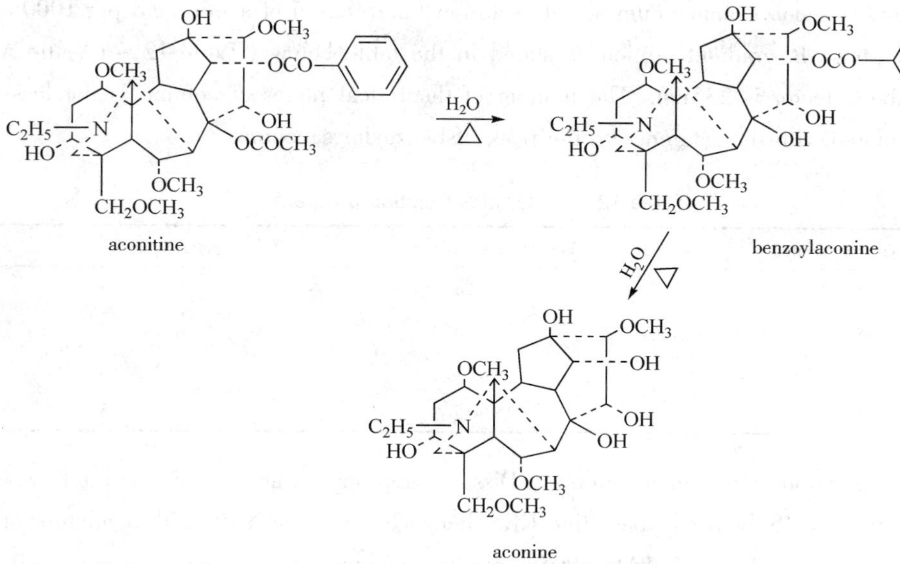

Fig. 12 – 1　Hydrolysis action of aconitine

Instruments and chemicals

1. Instruments

Boiler, pressure cooker, balance, funnel, HPLC, ultrasonic surge, microsyringe, micro – porous filtration member, 50ml conical flask with stopper, 50ml pipettes, 5ml pipettes.

2. Chemtcals

Benzoylaconitine CRS, benzoylhypacoitine CRS, benzoylmesaconine CRS, aconitine CRS, mesaconitine CRS, hypaconitine CRS, ammonia TS, acetonitrile (chromatographicial pure), tetrahydrofuran (chromatographicial pure), 0. 1mol/L ammonium acetate solution, acetic acid, isopropyl alcohol (chromatographicial pure), chloroform (chromatographicial pure), ethyl acetate.

Experiment contents

1. Boiling Method

(1) Processedaconite root: Take 100g of cleaned drugs, classify according to the size, and soak with water until the center of the drug is no longer hard, take out and boil with water (fully soaked the drugs) for 4 to 6 hours, or steam for 6 to 8 hours, or boil by pressure cooker for about 50 minutes until no white center appear, and taste slightly numb. Take out, slice and dry in the air or oven (for approximately 3 hours below 80℃).

(2) Characteristics of finished products: Blackish brown, crisp, odorless, taste slightly numb.

(3) Processing action: The raw aconite root is toxic, and mostly used externally, boiling can reduce the toxicity of the drug and can be used orally.

2. Assay of alkaloid

HPLC method

(1) Chromatographic system and system suitability: Use octadecylsilane bonded silica gel as the stationary phase, a mixture of acetonitrile – tetrahydrofuran (25∶15) as the mobile phase A, and 0.1mol/L ammonium acetate solution (add 0.5ml of acetic acid per 1000ml) as the mobile phase B, gradient elution as stated in the table below (Table 12 – 1); the wavelength of the detector is 235nm. The number of theoretical plates of column is not less than 2000, calculated with the reference to the peak of benzoylmesaconine.

Table 12 – 1   Gradient elution program

Time (minute)	mobile phase A (%)	mobile phase B (%)
0—48	15→26	85→74
48—48.1	26→35	74→65
48.1—58	35	65
58—65	35→15	65→85

(2) Preparation of reference solution: Dissolve appropriate amount of accurately weighed benzoylaconitine CRS, benzoylhypacoitine CRS, benzoylmesaconine CRS with a mixture of isopropyl alcohol – chloroform (1∶1) to obtain solution contains 20μg of benzoylaconitine, 0.1mg of benzoylhypacoitine and 80μg of benzoylmesaconine per ml.

(3) Preparation of test solution: Weighed accurately 2g of raw and processed aconite root powder, and put them into stopped concial flask separately, add 3ml of ammonia TS, and add 50ml of mixture of alcohol – ethyl acetate (1∶1) accurately, stopper tightly and weigh. Ultrasonicate (300W, 40kHz, water temperature is below 25℃) for 30 minutes, cool to ambient temperature and weigh again. Replenish the lost weight with mixture of alcohol – ethyl acetate (1∶1), mix well, filter, measure accurately 25ml of successive filtrate and recover solvent to dry under 40℃ by decompression, add accurately 3ml of mixture of alcohol – chloroform (1∶1) to dissolve the residue, filter and use the successive filtrate as the test solution.

Assay: Accurately inject 10μl each of the reference solution and the test solution, respectively, and assay.

The assay of diester type alkaloid is according to the chromatographic conditions and thepreparation method of the test solution above.

(4) Preparation of reference solution: Dissolve appropriate amount of accurately weighed aconitine CRS, mesaconitine CRS, hypaconitine CRS with a mixture of isopropyl alcohol – chloroform (1∶1) to obtain solution contains 30μg of aconitine, 10μg of mesaconitine and 50μg of hypaconitine per ml.

Assay: Accurately inject 10μl each of the reference solution and the test solution, respectively, and assay.

3. Experiment of the toxicity of the raw and processed aconite root

(1) Preparation of sample solution: Weigh accurately 20g of powder of raw and processed aconite root respectively, add 200ml of steamed water, and boil for 30min, filter, boil the residue with water for 2 times, filter again. Collect the filtrate and concentrate to 10% sample solution,

filter.

（2）Toxic emperiment：Divide randomly 40 little mice with the weight ranging from 18 to 22g to 2 groups，weigh and indicate respectively，and then intraperitoneally inject the sample solution of raw and pressed drugs（0.5ml/10g）. Observe for 2 hours and record the intoxication symptom，the time and the number of death.

Experimental records

（1）Record experimental result of assay of alkaloid and toxic emperiment.

（2）Make a record of the problems appeard during the experiment and explain the causes of the problems.

Matters needing attention

Pay attention to safety operation since aconite root is hypertoxic.

Questions

（1）What are the processing methods of aconite root? What is the similarities and differences of these processing methods?

（2）What is the purpose and principle of processing of aconite root?

实验十三　燀法及其对苦杏仁中苦杏仁苷的影响

【实验目的】

1. 掌握燀法的目的和注意事项。

2. 熟悉苦杏仁苷定性定量分析方法。通过定性定量分析，明确苦杏仁燀制的目的。

【实验原理】

燀法可以利于保存药物有效成分，去除非药用部位，或分离不同药用部位。

苦杏仁止咳平喘的有效成分是苦杏仁苷，易被共存的苦杏仁酶和野樱酶水解，产生氢氰酸而散逸（图13-1）。燀制可以杀酶保苷，有利于保存药效，降低毒性，并且燀制后便于去除种皮。

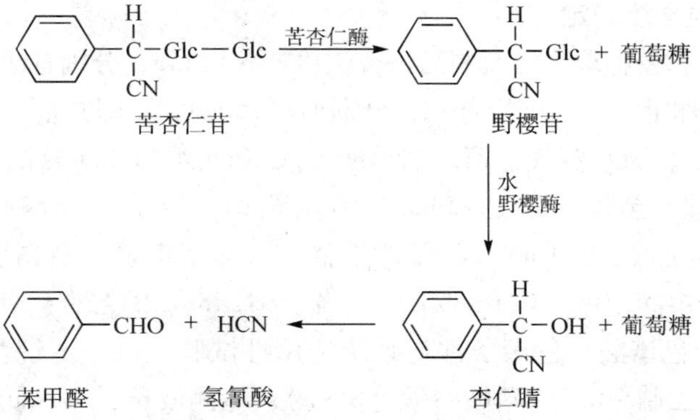

图13-1　苦杏仁苷的酶解反应

【实验器材】

1. 仪器 锅、漏勺、烧杯、天平、量筒、水浴锅、水蒸气发生器、试管、滤纸、漏斗、软木塞、凯氏烧瓶、冷凝装置、酸式滴定管、高效液相色谱仪、超声波清洗器、微量进样器、微孔滤膜、具塞锥形瓶、50ml 量瓶、5ml 移液管。

2. 试剂 苦杏仁苷标准品、碘化钾试液、碳酸钠试液、氢氧化钠试液、硫酸亚铁溶液、稀盐酸、三氯化铁试剂、氨试液、苦味酸（三硝基苯酚）试纸、0.1mol/L 硝酸银滴定液、甲醇（色谱纯）、乙腈（色谱纯）、0.1% 磷酸溶液。

【实验内容】

一、燀法

1. 苦杏仁 取净杏仁置 10 倍量沸水中略煮，加热约 10 分钟，至种皮微膨起即捞出，用凉水浸泡，取出，搓去种皮。

2. 成品性状 燀苦杏仁无种皮，乳白色，具特殊香气，味苦。

3. 炮制作用 加热燀制便于除去种皮，并可使酶灭活，以减少苦杏仁苷的酶解（杀酶保苷），提高药效，降低毒性。

二、苦杏仁生、燀品中苦杏仁苷的含量比较

1. 定性分析

（1）苦味酸钠试验 取生、制苦杏仁粗粉各约 0.5g，分别置试管中，加水数滴使润湿，在试管口悬挂一条用碳酸钠试液润湿过的苦味酸钠试纸，密塞，置 40℃ ~50℃ 的水浴中放置 15 分钟，生品中苦杏仁受酶的作用而水解，放出氢氰酸，接触苦味酸钠试纸，发生还原反应，生成异紫酸钠显砖红色，而制品则不显砖红色。

（2）普鲁士蓝试验 取生、制苦杏仁粗粉各约 0.2g，分别置小试管中，加水润湿，立即用氢氧化钠溶液润湿的滤纸将管口包紧，置 40℃ ~50℃ 的水浴中加热数分钟，在滤纸上加硫酸亚铁溶液 1 滴、稀盐酸 1 滴、三氯化铁试剂 1 滴，滤纸即显蓝色，为亚铁氰化铁。

2. 苦杏仁苷的含量测定

（1）滴定法 精密称取生品及制品苦杏仁粉末各约 15g，分别置凯氏烧瓶中，制品苦杏仁中再加入精密称定的苦杏仁粉末 4g，分别加水 150ml，立即密塞，置 37℃ 水浴中保温 2 小时，连接冷凝管，通水蒸气蒸馏，馏出液导入 10ml 水与 2ml 氨试液的吸收液中，接收瓶置冰浴中冷却，至馏出液达 60ml 时停止蒸馏，馏出液加碘化钾试液 2ml，用 0.1mol/L 硝酸银滴定液（0.1mol/L）液缓缓滴定，至溶液显出黄白色混浊不消失即为终点。每 1ml 硝酸银滴定液（0.1mol/L）相当于 91.48mg 的苦杏仁苷（$C_{20}H_{27}NO_{11}$）。

（2）高效液相色谱法 色谱条件与系统适用性试验：以十八烷基硅烷键合硅胶为填充剂；流动相：乙腈 -0.1% 磷酸溶液（8:92）；检测波长：207nm。理论板数按苦杏仁苷峰计算应不低于 7000。

对照品溶液的制备：取苦杏仁苷对照品适量，精密称定，加甲醇制成每 1ml 含

40μg 的溶液，即得。

供试品溶液的制备：取生、制苦杏仁粉末（过二号筛）约 0.25g，精密称定，置具塞锥形瓶中，精密加入甲醇 25ml，密塞，称定重量，超声处理（功率 250W，频率 50kHz）30 分钟，放冷，再称定重量，用甲醇补足减失的重量，摇匀，滤过，精密量取续滤液 5ml，置 50ml 量瓶中，加 50% 甲醇稀释至刻度，摇匀，滤过，取续滤液，即得。

测定法：分别精密吸取对照品溶液与供试品溶液各 10～20μl，注入液相色谱仪，测定，即得。

【实验记录】

（1）记录定性分析、苦杏仁苷的含量测定实验结果。

（2）记录实验中出现的问题并说明原因。

【注意事项】

（1）焯制时必须水沸后再投入药材，用水量为药材量 10 倍以上，时间为 5～10 分钟，时间太短则酶灭活不完全，时间过长易造成苦杏仁苷损失。

（2）含量测定要掌握高效液相色谱法和水蒸气蒸馏的装置和操作要点。测定时要避光，滴定时密切注意终点变化。

【思考题】

（1）苦杏仁焯制的目的是什么，焯制有哪些注意事项？

（2）苦杏仁苷定性定量的原理是什么？

Experiment 13   The Method of Scalding and its Influence on the Content of Amygdalin in Armeniacae Semen Amarum

Purpose

1. To master the purpose and notes of scalding method.

2. To familiarize with the method of qualitative and quantitative analysis of amygdalin, definitude the aim of processing bitter apricot kernel through qualitative and quantitative analysis of amygdalin.

Principle

Scalding method is facilitate to preserve effective component, remove the nonmedicinal part, or separate the different medicinal parts.

Armeniacae Semen Amarum contains amygdalin, which is the active constituent for relieving cough and asthma. Amygdalin can be enzymolyse by amygdalase and prunase to produce hydrocyanic acid (Fig. 13 – 1). Scalding can inactivate the enzyme to avoid the enzymatic hydrolysis of amygdalin and then enhance the clinical effect, reduce the toxicity, and be convenient for removing the seed coat.

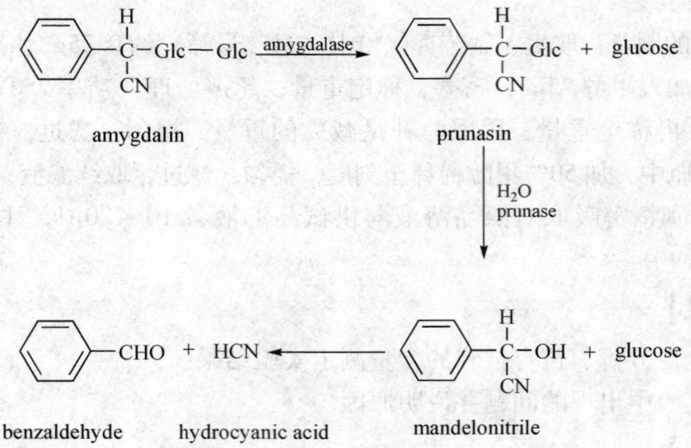

Fig. 13 - 1 Enzymolyse action of amygdalin

Instruments and chemicals

1. Instruments

Pan, colander, beaker, scales, measuring cylinder, water bath, steam generator, test tube, filter paper, funnel, cork, Kjeldahl flask, condensing unit, acid burette, HPLC, ultrasonic surge, microsyringe, microporous filtration member, conical flask with stopper, 50ml volumetric flask, 5ml pipettes.

2. Chemicals

Amygdalin CRS, potassium iodide TS, sodium carbonate TS, sodium hydroxide TS, ferrous sulfate TS, dilute hydrochloric TS, irontrichlorid TS, ammonia TS, picric acid (trinitrophenol) test paper, 0. 1mol/L silver nitrate VS, methanol (chromatographicial pure), acetonitrile (chromatographicial pure), 0. 1% phosphoric acid solution.

Experiment contents

1. Scalding Method

(1) Scalded Armeniacae Semen Amarum: Put the cleaned Armeniacae Semen Amarum into the boiling water which is about 10 times volume of that of the drugs, heat for about 10 minutes, take them out as the seed coats are expanded and soak in cold water. Take them out and separate the seed coat and kernel by rubbing.

(2) Characteristics of finished products: No seed coat, milk white, having special fragrance, taste bitter.

(3) Processing action: Heating to be convenient for removing the seed coat and inactivate the enzyme to avoid the enzymatic hydrolysis of amygdalin so as to enhance the clinical effect, reduce the toxicity.

2. Content of amygdalin in raw and scalded Armeniacae Semen Amarum

(1) Qualitative analysis

①Sodium picrate test: Weigh about 0. 5g of coarse powder of raw and scalded Armeniacae

Semen Amarum, put them into test tube separately, and add several drops of water to moist the powder. Hang a strip of picric acid test paper which has been wetted by sodium carbonate TS, and stopper tightly and heat for 15 minutes on water bath at 40℃ ~ 50℃, the amygdalin in the raw drug been enzymatic hydrolyze to release HCN which react with sodium picrate, and then the paper turns to brick - red color, while the paper of processed drug shows no obvious color change.

②Bronze blue test: Weigh about 0.2g of coarse powder of raw and scalded Armeniacae Semen Amarum, put them into test tube separately, and add several drops of water to moist the powder. Wrap up the mouth of tube tightly with filter paper which moistened by potassium hydroxide TS, and heat for several minutes on water bath at 40℃ ~ 50℃, add a drop of ferrous sulfate TS, dilute hydrochloric TS, and iron trichloride TS on the filter paper, and the filter paper turns to blue color, which is ferric ferrocyanide (Berlin blue).

(2) Quantitative analysis

①Titrimetry: Weigh accurately 15g of raw and scalded Armeniacae Semen Amarum powder and put them into kjeldahl flask separately, add 150ml of water and immediately stopper tightly, heat at 37℃ on water bath for 2 hours. Connect the condenser, distill and collect the distillate with receiver containing 10ml of water and 2ml of ammonia TS, and cool on ice bath until 60ml of distillate has been received. Add 2ml of potassium iodide TS in the distillate and titrate with silver nitrate (0.1mol/L) v. s. slowly until yellowish white turbid substance don't disappear. Each ml of silver nitrate (0.1mol/L) v. s. equals to 91.48mg of amygdalin ($C_{20}H_{27}NO_{11}$).

②HPLC method

Chromatographic system and system suitability: Use octadecylsilane bonded silica gel as the stationary phase and a mixture of acetonitrile - 0.1% solution of phosphoric acid (8∶92) as the mobile phase; the wavelength of the detector is 207nm. The number of theoretical plates of column is not less than 7000, calculated with the reference to the peak of amygdalin.

Preparation of reference solution: Dissolve appropriate amount of accurately weighed amygdalin CRS with ethanol TS to obtain solution contains 40μg of amygdalin per ml.

Preparation of test solution: Weighed accurately 0.25g of raw and scalded Armeniacae Semen Amarum powder, and put them into stopped concial flask separately, add 25ml of ethanol accurately, stopper tightly and weigh. Ultrasonicate (250W, 50kHz) for 30 minutes, cool to ambient temperature and weigh again. Replenish the lost weight with ethanol, mix well, filter and use the successive filtrate as the test solution.

Assay: Accurately inject 10 ~ 20μl each of the reference solution and the test solution, respectively, and assay.

Experimental records

(1) Record experimental result of qualitative analysis and quantitative analysis.

(2) Make a record of the problems appeard during the experiment and explain the causes of the problems.

Matters needing attention

(1) To scald the drug, the water must be boiling and then add the drug. The volume of wa-

ter must be above 10 times of that of the drug, and boil for 5 to 10 minutes. The enzyme inactivation is not complete if time is too short, and too long to cause loss of amygdalin.

(2) To master themain points of the installation and operation of HPLC method and the steam distillation method. Avoid light while determine, and pay close attention to the change at the end point.

Questions

(1) What are the processing action and the note of scalding the bitter apricot kernel?

(2) What is the principle of qualitative and quantitative analysis of amygdalin?

实验十四 复制法、煨法、结晶法、水飞法

【实验目的】

掌握复制法、煨法、结晶法、水飞法的炮制方法、目的和注意事项。

【实验原理】

复制法可以降低或消除药物毒性,改变药性,增强疗效,矫味矫臭。

煨法可以降低药物副作用,增强疗效,缓和药性。

结晶法可以使药物纯净,提高疗效,缓和药性,降低毒性。

水飞法可以洁净药物,使药物质地细腻,便于外用和内服,防止粉尘飞扬污染环境,并可除去药物中易溶于水的毒性成分。

【仪器器材】

1. 仪器 烧杯、量筒、乳钵、铁锅、铲子、天平、筛子、盆、玻璃棒、吸油纸、滤纸、漏斗、布氏漏斗、抽滤瓶。

2. 试剂 8%白矾溶液、甘草、生石灰、麦麸、面粉、滑石粉、萝卜。

【实验内容】

一、复制法

半夏的炮制

1. 清半夏 取净半夏,大小分开,用8%白矾溶液浸泡2~3日,至内无干心,口尝稍带麻舌感,取出,洗净,切厚片,干燥。

辅料用量:每100kg半夏,用白矾20kg。

成品性状:清半夏切面淡灰色至浅白色,质脆,气微,味微咸涩,微有麻舌感。

炮制作用:降低毒性,缓和药性,消除副作用。以燥湿化痰为主。

2. 姜半夏 取净半夏,大小分开,用水泡至内无干心(如起泡沫时加白矾适量),另取生姜切片煎汤,加白矾与半夏共煮透,取出,晾至半干,切薄片,干燥。

辅料用量:每100kg半夏,用生姜25kg,白矾12.5kg。

成品性状:姜半夏呈淡黄色片状,有角质样光泽,气微香,味辛辣,微有麻舌感。

炮制作用:降低毒性,缓和药性,消除副作用。以降逆止呕为主。

3. **法半夏** 取净半夏，大小分开，用水泡至内无干心，去水，加入甘草－石灰液（取甘草加适量水煎 2 次，合并煎液，倒入适量水制成的石灰液中）浸泡，每日搅拌 1~2 次，并保持 pH 12 以上，至口尝微有麻舌感，切面黄色均匀为度，取出，洗净，阴干或烘干。

辅料用量：每 100kg 半夏，用甘草 15kg、生石灰 10kg。

成品性状：黄色或淡黄色颗粒，气微，味淡略甘，微有麻舌感。

炮制作用：降低毒性，缓和药性，消除副作用。以祛寒痰为主。

二、煨法

（一）肉豆蔻的炮制

1. **面裹煨肉豆蔻** 取面粉加适量水做成面团，再压成薄片，将肉豆蔻逐个包裹，或将药物表面用水润湿，如水泛丸法包裹面粉 3~4 层，晾至半干，投入已炒热的滑石粉，适当翻动，煨至面皮呈焦黄色时取出，筛去滑石粉，放凉，剥去面皮，即得。

辅料用量：每 100kg 肉豆蔻，用面粉、滑石粉各 50kg。

2. **麦麸煨肉豆蔻** 取净肉豆蔻，与麦麸同置锅内，文火加热并适当翻动，至麦麸呈焦黄色，肉豆蔻呈深棕色时取出，筛去麦麸，放凉，即得。

辅料用量：每 100kg 肉豆蔻，用麦麸 40kg。

3. **滑石粉煨肉豆蔻** 先将滑石粉放入锅内加热至 120℃~140℃，呈灵活状态时再投入肉豆蔻，不断搅拌，以便受热均匀，至肉豆蔻表面附着一层较油润的滑石粉时，取出，筛去滑石粉，放凉。

辅料用量：每 100kg 肉豆蔻，用滑石粉 50kg。

成品性状：肉豆蔻煨后表面呈棕黄色或深棕色，显油润，香气更浓，味辛辣。

炮制作用：生肉豆蔻含大量油质，有滑肠之弊，且有刺激性；煨后去油免于滑肠，刺激性减小，增强了固肠止泻的功效。

（二）木香的炮制

纸煨木香：取未干燥的木香片，均匀地铺在吸油纸上，再加一层纸，再铺一层木香片，反复铺放数层，捆紧，放于温度较高的地方，烘煨至木香所含挥发油渗透到纸上，取出木香，放凉。

成品性状：煨后色泽变深，香气较弱。

炮制作用：生木香行气作用强；煨后实肠止泻作用增强。

三、结晶法

芒硝的炮制

先将净萝卜切成薄片，置锅内，加适量水煮约 20~30 分钟，滤过，取汁去杂质，再将皮硝投入萝卜液中继续加热，不断搅拌，使皮硝全部溶化，趁热倒入布氏漏斗抽滤，滤液倒入烧杯中，10℃ 左右结晶，待结晶完全后，捞出晶体，避风干燥。即为成品芒硝。

辅料用量：每100kg皮硝，用萝卜20kg，水量约为药量2倍。

成品性状：无色透明，结晶为针状，或马尾状。

炮制作用：炮制后可提高芒硝的纯净度，并增强润燥软坚、下气通肠的功效。

四、水飞法

滑石的炮制

取滑石粗粉，加水少量，研磨至细，再加适量清水搅拌，倒出上层混悬液，下沉部分再按上法反复操作数次，合并混悬液，静置沉淀，倒去上清液，将沉淀物晒干后再研细粉。

成品性状：滑石粉为白色或青白色粉末，质细腻，手捻有滑润感。

炮制作用：滑石水飞后使药物达到极细和纯净，便于内服外用。

【注意事项】

（1）复制法漂泡时间的长短应根据药材的质地、大小及季节来决定。生半夏有毒，应注意安全。

（2）煨肉豆蔻时，辅料的温度要适当，以免影响药物的质量。

（3）煨木香要将木香片单层分放于纸上，药与纸要贴紧，放温度较高处。

（4）制芒硝加水量不宜过多，使药物全部溶解即可，否则不易结晶。

（5）水飞时药物研磨前应破碎成粗颗粒；加水研磨时水量宜少，以能研成糊状为宜；加水搅拌时水量宜大，以便除去在水中溶解度小的有毒物质及杂质，搅拌后应适当静置，使粗颗粒下沉；干燥时以晾干为宜。

【思考题】

（1）半夏有哪些炮制方法？其临床作用有何不同？

（2）肉豆蔻、木香为什么要煨制？

（3）芒硝为什么要与萝卜水同煮？

（4）水飞法有哪些注意事项？

Experiment 14　The Method of Repeatedly Processing, the Method of Roasting, the Method of Purification and the Method of Refining Powder with Water

Purpose

To master the method and purpose and notes of repeatedly processing method, roasting method, purification method and refining powder with water method.

Principle

Repeatedly processing method can reduce or eliminate drug's toxicity, alter its property, strengthen the therapeutic effectiveness and rectify its terrible odor and fishy smell.

Roasting method can reduce the side effect of drug, improve therapeutic effectiveness, and moderate the drug's property.

Purification method can purify the drug and improve therapeutic effectiveness, moderate the drug's property, and reduce the toxicity.

Refining powder with water method can eliminate the impurities to purify the drug, make drug fine and smooth to facilitate externally and orally applying, prevent the drug powder from flying up to pollute the environment, and remove the water soluble toxic substance.

Instruments and chemicals

1. Instruments

Beaker, cylinder, mortar, iron pot, shovel, balance, sieve, basin, glass rod, oil absorbing paper, filter paper, funnel, Buchner funnel, suction flask。

2. Chemicals

8% alum solution, licorice root, quick lime, wheat bran, flour, talcum powder, radish.

Experiment contents

1. Repeatedly Processing Method

The processing of pinellia tuber

(1) Processed pinellia tuber (Qingbanxia): Separate the cleaned drugs according to their size. Soak the drug with 8% alum solution until the drug's center is no longer hard and taste slightly numb. Take them out and wash. Cut into slices and dry.

20kg of alum is used for every 100kg of pinellia tubers.

Characteristics of finished products: Section light gray to pale white, crisp, odorless, taste slightly salty, slightly numb.

Processing action: Reduce toxicity, transition resistance, eliminate side effects. Mainly used to removing dampness to reduce phlegm.

(2) Ginger – processed pinellia tuber (Jiangbanxia): Separate the cleaned drugs according to their size. Soak the drug with clean water until the drug's center is no longer hard (add appropriate amount of alum if the water froths). Put the drug into the decoction of the fresh ginger and add certain amount of alum, then boil them together thoroughly. Take out and dry to half dryness. Cut into slices and dry.

25kg of fresh ginger and 12. 5kg of alum are used for every 100kg of pinellia tubers.

Characteristics of finished products: Slightly yellow, slice form, horny like luster, slightly fragrant, taste pungent, slightly numb.

Processing action: Reduce toxicity, transition resistance, eliminate side effects. Mainly used to controlling nausea and vomiting.

(3) Pinellia tuber processed with several assistant materials (Fabanxia): Separate the cleaned drugs according to their size. Soak the drug with clean water until the drug's center is no longer hard. Put the drug into the mixed solution of the licorice root decoction and quick lime – water solution (decoct the licorice root with water for two times and add the decoction

into the lime – water solution), soak, and stir one or two times every day, keep pH value above 12, until the drug taste slightly numb and the cross section appears evenly yellow. Take out and wash, dry in the shade or oven.

15kg of licorice root and 10kg of quick lime are used for every 100kg of pinellia tubers.

Characteristics of finished products: Yellow or slightly yellow granules, odorless, slightly sweet, tasteless, slightly numb.

Processing action: Reduce toxicity, transition resistance, eliminate side effects. Mainly used to reducing phlegm caused by cold.

2. Roasting Method

The processing of nutmeg

(1) Roasted nutmeg covered with flour: Make the flour into dough with water and press it into thin piece. Wrap the nutmegs with the flour piece one by one. Or moisten the surface of the nutmegs with water and then make them roll in the flour like making wter – paste pill. Repeat the procedure for 3 ~ 4 times. Dry to half dryness, and put them in the hot talcum powder, stir – fry until the flour paste becomes scorched yellow. Take them out and sift out the talcum powder, cool and peel the flour paste.

50kg of flour and talcum powder are used for every 100kg of nutmegs.

(2) Nutmeg roasted in wheat bran: Put the nutmeg and wheat bran into the pot together, heat with soft fire and stir properly. Take them out while the wheat bran becomes scorched yellow and the nutmegs become dark brown. Sift out the wheat bran and cool.

40kg of wheat bran is used for every 100kg of nutmegs.

(3) Nutmeg roasted in talcum powder: Put the talcum powder in the pot and heat to make it to be smoothness (about 120℃ ~ 140℃). Then put the nutmegs in it, stir – fry until the nutmegs covered with a layer of oily talcum powder. Take out and sift out the talcum powder and cool.

50kg of flour and talcum powder is used for every 100kg of nutmegs.

Characteristics of finished products: Brownish yellow or dark brown, oily moist, aromatic, taste pungent.

Processing action: The raw nutmeg contains large amount of oil with laxative action and irritation, the processed nutmeg has less laxative action and irritation, and the effect of relieving diarrhea with astringents has been strengthened.

The processing of costus root

Costus root roasted in paper: Take the undried drug pieces, spread them on the oil absorbing paper, a layer of paper being alternating with a layer of drug pieces. Clip several layers like this and bundling them up tightly, and place them in the place with high temperature. Roast them until the volatile oil permeates the oil absorbing paper, then take the drug out and cool.

Characteristics of finished products: Brownish yellow, slightly fragrant.

Processing action: The raw costus root has strong effect of promoting the circulation of

Qi. The drug's effect of reinforcing intestine to stop diarrhea has been enhanced by processing.

3. Purification Method

The processing of mirabilite

Cut the cleaned fresh radish into pieces, and boil with water for 20—30 minutes, filter to get the solution. Put the natural mirabilite in the solution, heat and stir until the mirabilite dissolved. Transfer the hot solution into the Buchner funnel and suction filter. Put the filtrate in a beaker and recrystallize at low temperature (about 10℃). Separate the crystal and dry.

20kg of fresh radish are used for every 100kg of mirabilite. The weight of water is about twice of the drug's weight.

Characteristics of finished products: Colorless, transparent, needle or horsetail form crystal.

Processing action: Increase purity and strengthen the effects of moistening and softening digestion, keeping the adverse Qi flowing downward and relaxing the bowels.

4. Refining Powder with Water Method

The processing of talc

Take the coarse powder of talc, grind it into fine powder with a little water. Add large amount of water, stir, and pour out the suspension. Process the sunken sediment as the above procedure repeatedly. Collect the suspension and settle for some time. Pour out the upper layer clear water. Take the sediment and dry in the sun, grind into fine powder.

Characteristics of finished products: White or bluish white powder, fine and smooth.

Processing action: Make the drug pure and extremely fine to facilitate orally administrating and externally applying.

Matters needing attention

(1) During the processing of pinellia tuber, the soaking time determines by the temperature of circumstance and the texture and size of drug, and be careful since the pinellia tuber is toxic.

(2) When process nutmeg, stir – fry the drug at appropriate temperature.

(3) Put only one layer of costus root between oil absorbing paper, and make sure the drug is close to the paper and place at high circumstance temperature.

(4) Add not too much water to dissolve the mirabilite when processing, or it is difficult to recrystallization.

(5) When processing by method of refining powder with water, the drug should be broken into coarse particle before grinding. Add small amount of water when grinding, and add large amount of water when stirring, so that the toxic insoluble substances and impurities in water can be removed. Stand appropriately after stirring to sink the coarse particle. It is advisable to dry by airing, but not heating.

Questions

(1) How to process pinellia tuber? What is the clinical application of different products?

（2）What is the processing action of nutmeg and costus root?

（3）Why boil mirabilite with radish?

（4）What is the note of refining powder with water method?

实验十五　制霜法及巴豆制霜前后脂肪油的含量测定

【实验目的】

1. 了解巴豆霜中巴豆油含量与巴豆霜质量的关系。

2. 明确巴豆制霜的炮制原理。

【实验原理】

生巴豆毒性强烈，仅供外用，其毒性成分主要包含在巴豆油中，去油制霜后能去除大部分的脂肪油，从而降低毒性，缓和峻泻作用。

巴豆油不溶于水，易溶于有机溶剂，较理想的巴豆油提取溶剂有乙醚、石油醚等。

【实验器材】

1. 仪器　吸油纸、盆、蒸锅、压榨器、纱布、瓦罐、毛刷、索氏提取器、水浴锅、称量瓶、分析天平、蒸发皿、干燥器、滤纸、乳钵、量筒、脱脂棉。

2. 试剂　芒硝；无水乙醚、无水硫酸钠。

【实验内容】

一、制霜法

（一）巴豆的炮制

取净巴豆仁，碾成泥状，用2～3层草纸包严。再用纱布包一层，蒸热，用压榨器榨去油，使油分被草纸吸收，如此反复更换草纸和加热加压，至药物松散成粉末，不再粘结成饼，草纸上基本无油为止。

少量者，可将巴豆仁碾碎后，用数层粗纸包裹，烘热，压榨去油，换纸后再烘再榨，如此反复数次，至纸上不再出现油痕，药物松散成粉末，不再粘结成饼为度。

成品性状：巴豆霜含油量应为18%～20%，呈暗黄色粉末，性滞腻，松散微显油性，味辛辣。

炮制作用：本品生品有大毒，仅供外用；去油制霜后降低毒性，缓和其峻泻作用，可内服。

（二）西瓜霜的制备

取新鲜西瓜瓤切碎，放入不带釉的瓦罐内，一层西瓜、一层芒硝，将口封严，悬挂于阴凉通风处，约10～15日即自瓦罐外面析出白色结晶物，随析随用毛刷收集，至无结晶析出为止。

辅料用量：每100kg西瓜，用芒硝15kg。

成品性状：本品为白色结晶性粉末，味微咸。

炮制作用：西瓜能清热解暑，芒硝能清热泻火，两药合制增强清热泻火的功效。

二、巴豆及巴豆霜的脂肪油含量测定

精密称取巴豆粉末约 1g、巴豆霜约 5g，分别装入滤纸筒内，上下均塞脱脂棉，置干燥索氏提取器中，由提取管上加入无水乙醚 100ml，水浴加热回流提取 6～8 小时，至脂肪油提尽，收集提取液，置已干燥至恒重的蒸发皿中，水浴上低温蒸干，在 100℃ 干燥 1 小时，移至干燥器中，冷却 30 分钟，精密称定，计算，即得。

$$巴豆油百分含量 = （巴豆油重/样品重）\times 100\%$$

【实验记录】

（1）记录巴豆油的量，填入表格。

（2）记录巴豆霜、西瓜霜的成品性状。

（3）记录实验中出现的问题并说明原因。

【注意事项】

（1）制备巴豆霜要注意劳动保护，应戴口罩手套；实验完毕用冷水洗手及用具；药材需加热才能有效去油；操作过程中要勤换纸；用过的纸和纱布要及时烧毁。

（2）制备西瓜霜应选在秋季凉爽有风时进行；瓦罐不可带釉；析出的霜应及时扫净。

（3）加入乙醚量不得超过烧瓶的 2/3。

（4）挥发乙醚时水浴温度以 40℃ 为宜，温度太高易溢出。

（5）乙醚易燃易爆，操作过程应避免明火。

【思考题】

（1）巴豆为什么要制霜炮制，有哪些注意事项？

（2）巴豆霜的质量由哪些方面进行控制？

Experiment 15　The Method of Frosting and the Assay of the Fatty Oil of Raw Crotonis Fructus and Frost of Crotonis Fructus

Purpose

1. To learn about the relations of the content of the fatty oil to the quality of the raw Crotonis Fructus and frost of Crotonis Fructus.

2. To master the process principle of FructusCrotonis.

Principle

The raw croton fruit is hypertoxic, and can be only used externally. The fatty oil is the main toxic component of the drug, and frosting by defatting can remove most fatty oil to reduce

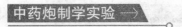

toxicity and moderates purgative action.

The fatty oil is insoluble in water and easy to solve in organic solvent, the best solvent are petrolic ether and ether.

Instruments and chemicals

1. Instruments

Oil absorbing paper, basin, steamer, squeezer, gauze, unglazed crock, brush, Soxhlet extractor, water bath pot, weighing bottle, analytical balance, evaporating dish, desiccator, filter paper, measuring cylinder, absorbent cotton.

2. Chemicals

Mirabilite; Anhydrous diethyl ether, anhydrous sodium sulfate.

Experiment content

1. The method of frosting

The processing of Crotonis Fructus

Take the cleaned Crotonis Fructus and grind into a paste. Wrap it with 2 or 3 layers of oil absorbing paper and gauze in the outer layer. Heat and squeeze to defat it, then change the oil absorbing paper and gauze. Repeat the procedures until the drug becomes loose powder and it is no longer coherent, and the oil absorbing paper absorb no more oil.

To processing small amount of drug, grind it into a paste and wrap it with several layers of oil absorbing paper, heat and squeeze to defat it, then change the oil absorbing paper and gauze and repeat the procedures until the drug becomes loose powder and it is no longer coherent, and the oil absorbing paper absorb no more oil.

Characteristics of finished products: Frost of Crotonis Fructus contains 18% ~20% of fatty oil, and being dark yellow powder, greasy, oily, taste pungent.

Processing action: The raw is hypertoxic, and can be only used externally. Frosting by defatting can reduce its toxicity and moderates its purgative action, and can be used internally.

The preparation of frosted watermelon

Take the fresh watermelon, smash it and put into the unglazed crock, placing one layer of watermelon alternating with one layer of mirabilite. Seal the crock and hang it at a ventilated dark cool place for about 10 to 15 days. The white crystals separate out on the surface of the crock, collect the crystals with brush as they separate out until no more crystals separating.

15kg of mirabilite is used for every 100kg of watermelon.

Characteristics of finished products: White crystal powder, slightly salty.

Processing action: Watermelon has the effect of clearing away summer heat and the mirabilite has the effect of clearing heat and purging fire. When processed together, the drugs act cooperatively to strengthen the effects of clearing heat and purging fire.

2. The assay of the fatty oil of raw croton kernel and frost of Crotonis Fructus

Weigh accurately 1g of powder of raw Crotonis Fructus and 5g of frost of croton kernel, separately. And put in to two prepared filter paper tanks which have proper amount of absorbent cotton at the bottom and top of the tank. Put the filter paper tank into the Soxhlet extractor, and add 100ml of anhydrous diethyl ether, heat under reflux for 6 to 8 hours to extract fatty oil. Collect and remove the ether into a weighed evaporating dish (dry to constant weight), and heat at a low temperature to volatilize the ether. Dry the residue at 100℃ for 1 hour, cool for 30 minutes in desiccator, and weigh accurately. Calculate the content of the fatty oil in drugs.

Content of the fatty oil (%) = (the weight of fatty oil/ the weight of sample) × 100%

Experimental records

(1) Record the weight of fatty oil.

(2) Record the character of frosted watermelon and frost of croton kernel.

(3) Make a record of the problems appeard during the experiment and explain the causes of the problems.

Matters needing attention

(1) Wear gloves and gauze mask for protection when processing croton fruit, and wash hands and instruments with cold water after the operation. The drug needs heating to defatting effectively. The oil absorbing paper should be change frequently to remove oil. The used paper and gauze must be burned immediately after the operation.

(2) The apt time toprocess frosted watermelon is in autumn. The crock should not be glazed. Sweep the crystal in time.

(3) The amount of ether should not beyond 2/3 of the flask.

(4) The temperature of the water bath should be about 40℃ to avoid the loss of ether.

(5) Sinceether is flammable and explosive, the operation process should avoid open flames.

Questions

(1) What is the purpose of processing croton fruit by frosting by defatting? What is the master needing attention of the operation?

(2) How to control the quality of frost of Crotonis Fructus?

实验十六 中药六神曲发酵炮制工艺及质量评价

【实验目的】

1. 掌握固体发酵罐操作方法、发酵条件及成品发酵程度的控制方法。

2. 了解影响发酵的因素及药性的变化。

3. 明确发酵的目的和意义。

【实验原理】

中药发酵是将净制或处理后的药物，在一定的温度、湿度等环境条件下，借助于酶和微生物的催化、分解作用，使药物发泡、生衣的炮制方法。六神曲是传统的中药发酵品之一，是由面粉、麦麸、杏仁、赤小豆、鲜青蒿、鲜辣蓼、鲜苍耳草等原料配伍后发酵制成，具有健脾开胃功效。蛋白酶、淀粉酶的酶活力是检测六神曲发酵程度及其质量控制的重要指标。

【实验器材】

1. 仪器 DL－CJ－1N 超净工作台、多标记酶标仪、固态样品发酵罐、抑菌圈自动测量分析仪、温度梯度培养箱、水浴锅、锥形瓶、容量瓶、紫外分光光度仪等。

2. 药材及试剂 面粉、麦麸、杏仁、赤小豆、鲜青蒿、鲜辣蓼、鲜苍耳、蒸馏水、2%淀粉液、磷酸－柠檬酸缓冲液、比色稀碘液、酪氨酸、盐酸、碳酸钠、福林试液、酪蛋白、三氯乙酸等。

【实验内容】

一、自然发酵法制备六神曲的传统工艺

1. 处方 面粉 400g，麦麸 600g，杏仁、赤小豆各 40g，鲜青蒿、鲜辣蓼、鲜苍耳草各 70g。药汁为鲜草汁和其药渣煎出液。

2. 制法

（1）药料的粉碎和拌匀 将杏仁、赤小豆研成粉末，与面粉及麦麸拌匀。

（2）拌曲 将上述混合粉置容器内，陆续加入鲜青蒿、鲜苍耳草、鲜辣蓼压榨出的鲜汁，残渣加水煎汁，合并药液（约占原药量的 25%～30%）拌匀，搓揉成粗颗粒状，以手握成团，掷之即散为准。

（3）成形 将上述拌匀的药料（粗颗粒状），置发酵罐中，控制温度在 30℃，调节相对湿度 70%～80%，发酵时间为 7 日。

（4）发酵完成后，取出，成品切 2.5cm³ 块，干燥，即可。

二、酶活力的测定

1. 淀粉酶活力的测定 分别取上述工艺制备的六神曲样品及未发酵品（取六神曲原料，混匀，低温冷藏，备用），过筛，各取 10g 粉末，置 100ml 锥形瓶中，加入 100ml 蒸馏水，在 40℃的恒温水浴锅中保温 1 小时，取出，离心，取上清液，即得六神曲样品的酶液。再取 9 个试管依次编号，分别加入 5ml 2%淀粉液和 0.5ml pH 6.0 磷酸－柠檬酸缓冲液，在 60℃水浴锅中预热 5 分钟后，分别加入 10ml 已预热的六神曲样品酶液，迅速混匀，即反应开始，记下时间 T_1。根据预实验结果，每隔一定时间吸取 1ml 反应液，注入预先装有 3ml 比色稀碘液的试管中，摇匀后与标准比色管比较，当与标准比色管色度相同时即为反应终点，再记下时间 T_2，两次时间间隔即为反应时间。

按公式计算，淀粉酶活力 =（60/t）×5×2%×10/10 = 6/t（t 为完成反应所需时间）。

2. 蛋白酶活力测定

（1）标准曲线绘制 酪氨酸在 105℃干燥至恒重，精确称取 0.1g，加入 HCl 使溶解，加蒸馏水定容至 1000ml，取 10ml 容量管 6 只，分别加入酪氨酸溶液 0、2、4、6、8、10ml，加蒸馏水至刻度。另取 6 只试管，编号 1～6，依次加入不同浓度的酪氨酸溶

液 1ml，再分别加 0.4mol/L 碳酸钠 5ml，福林试液 1ml，蒸馏水 2ml，摇匀置于水浴锅中，40℃恒温 20 分钟。于 680nm 波长处测定，测 3 次，取平均值，将 2～6 号管所测吸光度减去 1 号管的吸光度得实测值 A，以 A 为纵坐标，酪氨酸的浓度（C）为横坐标，得到回归方程。

（2）样品测定　取上述两种工艺制备的六神曲样品及原料各 1g，过筛，研细，加蒸馏水 20ml，于 40 ℃水浴放置 1 小时，间断搅拌，过滤，滤液以磷酸钠缓冲液稀释 1 倍。取 1ml 稀释液加至离心管，于 40℃水浴预热 5 分钟，加入预热的酪蛋白 1ml，精确保温 10 分钟，立即加入 0.4mol/L 三氯乙酸 2ml，终止反应，继续置水浴中保温 20 分钟，使残余蛋白质沉淀后离心滤过。取 1ml 滤液加至试管，加 0.4mol/L 碳酸钠 5ml，福林试液 1ml，蒸馏水 2ml，摇匀保温发色 20 分钟，于 680nm 波长测光吸收度。另取 1 只离心管作为空白对照，先加入 2ml 三氯乙酸，使酶失活，再加入酪蛋白，其余同前。每份样品测定 3 次。在 40℃时每 1 分钟水解酪蛋白产生 1μg 酪氨酸的酶量，定义为 1 个蛋白酶活力单位。测定结果列于表中。

（3）将固态样品发酵罐、温度梯度培养箱中的发酵成品进行比较，分析。

3. **菌种检测**　利用抑菌圈自动测量分析仪，检测成品菌种，并对固态样品发酵罐、温度梯度培养箱中的发酵成品进行比较，分析。

三、成品性状检测

六神曲为立方形小块，表面灰黄色，粗糙，质脆易断，微有香气。

【实验记录】

（1）记录六神曲性状、酶活力测定结果。

（2）记录成品菌种。

（3）记录实验中出现的问题并说明原因。

【注意事项】

（1）发酵过程要保证一定温度与湿度。

（2）注意仪器使用方法。

【思考题】

发酵前后六神曲消化酶活力有何不同？

Experiment 16　The Processing Technology and Quality Evaluation of Massa Medicata Fermentata （Comprehensive Experiment）

Purpose

1. To master the operation of solid fermenting equipment, and to master the control methods of the fermenting conditions and fermenting degree of the fermented product.

2. To understand the influencing factors of fermentation and the change of drug.

3. To know the purpose and significance of fermentation.

Principle

Fermentation of TCM is the method of making cleaned or treated drugs bubbling and covering due to the catalysis and decomposition of mold and enzyme under the condition of a certain temperature and humidity. Massa Medicata Fermentata is produced by fermenting Flour , wheat bran , red bean , bitter almond , fresh herba artemisiae annuae , fresh Polygonum hydropiper , and fresh Xanthium sibiricum. It has the function of strengthening spleen and stomach. The determination of enzyme activity (amylase activity and protease activity) is an important method to control fermenting conditions and fermenting degree.

Instruments and chemicals

1. Instruments

DL – CJ – 1N clean bench , ELIASA , solid fermenting equipment , automaticinhibition zone analyzer , temperature gradient incubator , water bath , conical flask , volumetric flask , ultraviolet spectrophotometry , etc.

2. Chemicals

Flour , wheat bran , red bean , bitter almond , fresh herba artemisiae annuae , fresh Polygonum hydropiper , fresh Xanthium sibiricum , distilled water , 2% starch solution , pH6. 0 phosphoric acid – citric acid buffer solution , colorimetric dilute iodine solution , tyrosine , hydrochloric acid , sodium carbonate , Folin solution , casein , TCA , etc.

Experimental Contents

1. The traditional technology of fermented Massa Medicata Fermentata

(1) Prescription : Flour 400g , wheat bran 600g , red bean 40g , bitter almond 40g , fresh herba artemisiae annuae 70g , fresh Polygonum hydropiper 70g , fresh Xanthium sibiricum 70g. Fresh Chinese traditional drugs' juice and dregs of a decoction product physic liquor.

(2) Method

The crush and mix of medicinal materials : Grinding bitter almond and red bean into powder then mix well with flour and wheat bran.

Mixing : Take fresh herba artemisiae annuae , fresh Polygonum hydropiper and fresh Xanthium sibiricum. Add in water , decoct for 2 times , filtration and make liquid medicine concentrate to 25% ~ 30% of the drug material quanlity , then mix well with the above mixing powder. Rub the mixture until they can clump together and loose easily.

Fermentation : Put the mixture (coarse powder) we made earlier into solid fermenting equipment , heat sterilization at 30°C , relative humidity for 70% ~ 80% , and ferment for 7days.

After the fermentation , take out them and cut into slices of 2. 5 per cubic centimeter , and dry.

2. The determination of enzyme activity

(1) The determination of amylase activity : Weigh 10g of Massa Medicata Fermentata and crude drug powder (pass through sieves) , respectively , to a 100ml conical flask , adding in 100ml distilled water. Put the conical flask in the 40°C water bath , and stand for 1 hour , then centrifuge. Take the supernatant, that is the enzyme of shenqu. Then take 9 tubes and numbered consecutively, add 5ml of 2% starch solution and 5ml of pH 6. 0 phosphoric acid – citric acid buffer solution separately. Take the tubes in 60℃ water bath and stand for 5 minutes. Measure accurately 10ml of preheated Shenqu enzyme, and mix well rapidly. Write down the time T_1, which means staring of the chemical changes. According to the results of preliminary experiment, take 1ml of the mixture into the tube which including 3ml of colorimetric dilute iodine solution at regular intervals. Mix well and compared standard colorimetric tube until the same color with the standard's one, we call it the reaction endpoint T_2.

According to the formula to calculate: The determination of amylase activity = (60 / t) × 5 × 2% × 10 / 10 = 6 / t (t = T_2 – T_1)。

(2)The determination of protease activity

Preparation of standard curve: Weigh accurately 0. 1g tyrosine (dry to constant weight under 105℃)to 1000ml volumetric flask and dissolve in hydrochloric acid, then dilute with distilled water to volume. Measure accurately tyrosine solution 0, 2, 4, 6, 8 and 10ml, respectively, into 10ml volumetric flask and dilute with distilled water to volume. Then take 6 tubes and numbered consecutively, add 1ml of different concentrations tyrosine solution in turn. After above, add 5ml of 0. 4 mol/L sodium carbonate, 1ml of Folin solution and 2ml distilled water. Mix well. Put tubes in 40℃ water bath and stand for 20 minutes. Measure the absorbance at 680nm for 3 times and take the average. A means the absorbance of No. 2—6 minus the absorbance of No. 1. Take A as ordinate and the concentration of tyrosine as abscissa and plot the standard curve.

Sample assay: Weigh 1g of Massa Medicata Fermentata and crude drug powder (pass through sieves), respectively, add 20ml distilled water to the tube. Put the tube in the 40℃ water bath, and stand for 1 hour, intermittent mixing and then filter. Filtrate dilute with phosphate buffer to 1 times. Take 1ml diluent to centrifuge tube . Put the centrifuge tube in the 40℃ water bath and keeps 5 minutes, adding 1ml of preheating casein . After 10 minutes, add 2ml of 0. 4mol/L trichloroacetic acid immediately. Keep warm in water bath for 20 minutes, then centrifuge. Take 1ml filtrate into tube, adding 5ml of 0. 4mol/L sodium carbonate, 1ml of Folin solution and 2ml distilled water, mixing well and keep warm for 20 minutes. Measure the absorbance at 680nm for 3 times. Take the other centrifuge tube as vacancy, which adding 2ml TCA, casein and the others same above. A unit of protease activity means casein product 1μg enzyme of tyrosine per minutes at 40℃. The results listed in table.

The results of the drugs fermented in the solid fermenting equipment compare with the fermentation made in the temperature gradient incubator.

(3)Bacteria detection: Use automatic inhibition zone analyzer to detect bacteria . Analyze the different bewteen the drugs fermented in the solid fermenting equipment and the fermentation made in the temperature gradient incubator.

3. Charater analysis

Massa Medicata Fermentata is pieces of small cube, yellow – white clothes, rough, crisp and aroma.

Experimental records

（1）Record the Character of Massa Medicata Fermentata and determination of enzyme activity.

（2）Record the Bacteria.

（3）Make a record of the problems appeard during the experiment and explain the causes of the problems.

Matters needing attention

（1）Keeps the stable temperature and humidity of fementation.

（2）To master the operation of equipment.

Reflection Questions

What is the difference of digestive enzyme activity bewteen Shenqu and crude drugs?

实验十七　　发酵对淡豆豉中异黄酮的影响

【实验目的】

1. 掌握淡豆豉中异黄酮质量控制方法。

2. 了解影响淡豆豉发酵的因素及成品发酵的程度。

3. 明确淡豆豉发酵的目的和意义。

【实验原理】

淡豆豉是一味常用的传统中药，记载于《中国药典》，淡豆豉为豆科植物大豆的成熟种子，配以桑叶、青蒿发酵而成。具有解表、除烦、宣发郁热等功效，用于感冒、寒热头痛、烦躁胸闷、虚烦不眠等。

淡豆豉中主要的活性成分为异黄酮（染料木素、染料木苷、大豆苷元、大豆苷、黄豆黄素、黄豆黄苷），异黄酮对多种疾病包括肿瘤、心血管疾病、骨质疏松症和神经退行性疾病等发挥预防和治疗作用。

本实验通过 HPLC 法和 UV 法同时测定淡豆豉中异黄酮、大豆苷元和染料木素含量的方法，通过对样品的含量测定，说明淡豆豉炮制的意义。

【实验器材】

1. **仪器**　高效液相色谱仪（Agilent 1100），紫外检测器（Agilent Dual λ Absorbance Detector），UV－2550 紫外－可见分光光度计（日本岛津公司），色谱柱（Agilent HC－C18 4.6×250mm），电子分析天平（AG135），水浴锅，锥形瓶，容量瓶等。

2. **药材及试剂**　桑叶、青蒿、黑豆、染料木素、大豆苷元、乙醇、乙酸乙酯、甲醇－0.1% 冰醋酸水溶液（50∶50）。

【实验内容】

一、淡豆豉制法

取桑叶、青蒿各 70～100 g，加水煎煮，滤过，煎液拌入净大豆 1000g 中，俟吸尽后，蒸透，取出，稍晾，再置容器内，用煎过的桑叶、青蒿渣覆盖，闷使发酵至黄衣上遍时，取出，除去药渣，洗净，置容器内再闷 15~20 日，至充分发酵、香气溢出时，取出，略蒸，干燥，即得。

二、紫外-可见分光光度法测定异黄酮的含量结果

1. 对照品溶液的制备　精密称取染料木素对照品适量，用乙醇溶解并稀释成每 1ml 含有 72.0μg 的溶液，作为对照品溶液。

2. 标准曲线的制备　精密吸取染料木素对照品溶液 1.0ml、2.0ml、3.0ml、4.0ml、5.0ml 置 50ml 的量瓶中，用乙醇稀释到刻度，摇匀，按照紫外-可见分光光度法（《中国药典》）。在 261nm 处测定吸收度，以浓度为横坐标，吸收度为纵坐标，绘制标准曲线。

3. 测定法　取本品粉末约 0.5g，精密称定，置具塞锥形瓶中，精密加入稀乙醇 20ml，称定重量，超声处理 50 分钟，取出，放冷，再称定重量，用稀乙醇补足减失的重量，摇匀，滤过，精密吸取续滤液 5ml 置蒸发皿中，水浴蒸干，用 15ml 水定量转移置分液漏斗中，用乙酸乙酯 25ml 萃取 6 次，合并萃取液水浴蒸干，用乙醇溶解并稀释至 25ml 的量瓶中，摇匀，精密吸取 3ml 置 10ml 量瓶中，用乙醇稀释至刻度，摇匀，依法测定吸收度，计算，即得。

三、高效液相色谱法测定大豆苷元和染料木素的含量结果

1. 色谱条件　以十八烷基硅烷键合硅胶为填充剂，以甲醇-0.1% 冰醋酸水溶液（50:50）为流动相，检测波长为 261nm，流速为 1ml/min。

2. 对照品溶液的制备　分别精密称取大豆苷元和染料木素对照品适量，用甲醇溶解并稀释成每 1ml 分别含大豆苷元和染料木素 10.3μg 和 9.92μg 的溶液，作为对照品溶液。

3. 供试品溶液的制备　取本品粉末约 0.5g，精密称定，置具塞锥形瓶中，精密加入稀乙醇 20ml，称定重量，超声处理 50 分钟，取出，放冷，再称定重量，用稀乙醇补足减失的重量，摇匀，滤过，取续滤液，即得。

4. 测定法　分别精密吸取对照品溶液与供试品溶液各 10μl，注入液相色谱仪，测定，即得。

【实验记录】

（1）记录紫外-可见分光光度法测定、高效液相色谱法测定大豆苷元和染料木素的数据。

（2）记录实验中出现的问题并说明原因。

【注意事项】

发酵过程要保证一定的温度与湿度。

【思考题】

发酵前后异黄酮有何不同？

Experiment 17   Comparative Studies on the Isoflavones Between the Crude and Semen Sojae Preparatrm

Purpose

1. To master the methods of quality control about SSP.

2. To understand the influencing factors of fermentation and thedegree of fermentation of the fermented product.

3. To know the purpose and significance of SSP's fermentation.

Principle

Semen Sojae Preparatrm is a famous traditional Chines medicine obtained by fermentation from Soybean, Folium Mori and Herba Artemisiae Annuae and officially listed in the Chinese Pharmacopoeia. With the action of diaphoresis, relieving restlessness, and dispelling emission heat. It has been used to treat flu, headache, fidgeting due to deficiency and insomnia, etc.

The major active constituents of Semen Sojae Preparatrm are considered to be the isoflavones genistein, fenistin, daidzein, daidzin, glycitein and glycitin. Pharmacological tests revealed isoflavones have both weak estrogenic and weak antiestrogenic effects, and may also have the antioxidant, antidipsotropic, anticarcinogenic, antiatherogenic and antiosteoporotic activities, and have been used to treat tumors, osteoporosis, and so on.

In our experiments, using HPLC and UV methods to determine the content of isoflavones, such as Daidzein and Genistein. Detect the content of sample, then to explain the meaning of processing.

Instruments and Chemicals

1. Instruments

HPLC(Agilent 1100), UV – detector(Agilent Dual λAbsorbance Detector), UV – VIS spectrophotometer (SHIMADZU), chromatographic column (Agilent HC – C18 4.6 × 250mm), electronic analytical balance (AG135), volumetric flask, conical flask, water bath, etc.

2. Chemicals

Soybean, Folium Mori, Herba Artemisiae Annuae, genistein, daidzein, ethanol, ethyl acetate, methanol – 0.1% glacial acetic acid(50:50), etc.

Experimental Contents

1. Processing

Weigh Folium Mori and Herba Artemisiae Annuae 70 ~ 100g separately. Add in water and decoct. Filter and liquid medicine, then mix in 1000g soybean. Absorb completely and steam. Take out and cool a little. Cover soybean with dregs of decotion of Folium Mori and Herba Artemisiae Annuae, then put them in the incubator. Ferment for 6 ~ 8 days until "yellow clothes" overgrow, then take out and remove dregs of decoction. Wash cleanly and dry. Put them in the incubator that closed tightly for 15 ~ 20 days. Take out and steam, then to dryness.

2. UV method for the determination of isoflavones

(1) Reference standard solution preparation: Precisely take appropriate amounts of Genistein and put it into ethanol to make it containing 72.0μg Genistein per milliliter solution.

(2) Standard curve preparation: Precisely take 1.0ml, 2.0ml, 3.0ml, 4.0ml, 5.0ml Genistein reference standard solution and put them into 50ml volumetric flask. Add in ethanol to solve the residue and dilute to scale, and shake up evenly. Use UV method to determine the absorption value at 261nm. Take the absorbance as ordinate and the concentration as abscissa and plot the standard curve.

(3) Determination: Take 0.5g of the powder, weigh accurately, add ethanol 20ml, stopper, and weigh. Supersonic extraction for 50 minutes, take out. Add ethanol to the original weight, mixing well, and then filter. Precisely draw 5ml extracting solution, put it into a evaporating dish, and make it dry. Add up 15ml water to solve the residue, and extract with acetidin from water solution 6 times, and toties quoties 25ml. then combine acetidin layer, and make it dry, add up ethanol to solve the residue into 25ml volumetric flask and dilute to scale, and mix well, then precisely draw 3ml into 10ml volumetric flask and dilute to scale, and shake up evenly, to determine the absorption value with UV method, stand by.

3. HPLC method for the determination of Daidzein and Genistein

(1) Chromatographic conditions: 18 - alkyl - silane bonded silica was used as filler and methanol - 0.1% glacial acetic acid(50:50) as the mobile phase, the detection wavelength is 261nm, and the flow rate is 1ml/min.

(2) Reference standard solution preparation: Take appropriate amounts of Daidzein and Genistein reference substance precisely and put them into MeOH to make it containing 10.3μg and 9.92μg Daidzein and Genistein per milliliter solution respectively.

(3) Test solution preparation: Take the 0.5g powder of SSP precisely and put them into erlenmeyer flask, precisely add in 20ml 50% ethanol and weighting. Take ultrasound for 50 minutes and take out, then add ethanol to the original weight. Shake up evenly and filtration.

(4) Determination: Draw the test solution and control solution 10μl respectively, inject into HPLC to determine the content.

Experimental records

(1) Record experimental result of UV method for the determination of isoflavones and HPLC method for the determination of Daidzein and Genistein.

(2) Make a record of the problems appeard during the experiment and explain the causes of the problems.

Matters needing attention

Keep stable temperature and humidity in the course of fementation.

Reflection Questions

What is the difference of isoflavone bewteen SSP and crude drugs?

实验十八　综合设计实验

【实验目的】

1. 了解中药延胡索、马钱子、槐米的炮制方法。

2. 分别设计中药延胡索、马钱子、槐米不同炮制品中有效成分的定性、定量测定方法，通过分析炮制对有效成分的影响，加深对中药炮制作用的理解。

3. 提高查阅文献、综合运用专业知识的能力。

【实验内容】

（1）设计槐米不同炮制品中有效成分的含量测定方法。

（2）设计马钱子不同炮制品中有效成分的含量测定方法。

（3）设计延胡索不同炮制品中有效成分的含量测定方法。

【注意事项】

（1）实验设计内容完整。

（2）实验设计要求科学、合理、方法先进。

Experiment 18　Comprehensive Design Experiment

Purpose

1. To understand the processing method of Rhizoma Corydalis, semen strychni and Flos Sophorae.

2. To design qualitative and quantitative method of effective constituent of Rhizoma Corydalis, semen strychni and Flos Sophorae. Understand the processing effect deeply through Comparasion on the effective constituent contenets.

3. Improve the capacity of consulting literature and using specialty comprehensively.

Experimental Contents

（1）To design qualitative and quantitative method of effective constituent of Rhizoma Corydalis. Understand the processing effect deeply through comparasion on the effective constituent contenets.

（2）To design qualitative and quantitative method of effective constituent of semen strychni. Understand the processing effect deeply through comparasion on the effective constituent contenets.

（3）To design qualitative and quantitative method of effective constituent of Flos Sophorae. Understand the processing effect deeply through comparasion on the effective constituent contenets.

Matters needing attention

（1）The experimental design must be integrated.

（2）The content of experimental design must be scientific, reasonable and advanced.

附录　中药炮制实验常用术语

Appendix　General Term for TCM Processing

一、饮片净制相关术语

去根　remove the root（of herbal medicines）

去茎　remove the stem（of herbal medicines）

去茎叶　exclude the stem and leaves（of herbal medicines）

去枝梗　remove leaf stalk and twigs（of herbal medicines）

去刺　remove the thorn（of herbal medicines）

去粗皮　scrap off the coarse layer of bark（of herbal medicines）

去残肉　remove the fresh remained on animal bone or turtle shell

去翅　remove the wings of animal medicines

去核（免滑）　remove the core（for avoiding sliding）

去瓤（免胀）　remove the pulp（for avoiding distending）

去芦（免吐）　remove the residue of rhizome（for avoiding vomit）

去皮（免损气）remove the skin（for avoiding tremendous loss）

去心（免烦）　remove the core　or remove the plumule from seed（for avoiding fidget）

去鳞片　remove the scale or bud scale

去木心　remove the woody core of root（of herbal medicines）

去皮　remove the skin

去皮尖　remove the seed coat and radicle

去皮壳　remove peel or husk of herbal medicines

去头尾足翅　remove the head，tail，elytra，wings and legs of beetle

去壳　remove the outer skin

去须根　remove the fibrous root of herbal medicines

抢水洗　quick washing with large volume of water

菊花筛　mesh whose diameter about 15—20mm

发汗　moisture transmitted to the surface of drug by piling up

刮去青皮（竹）　scrap off the outer layer（of bamboo）

刮去外层粗皮　scrap off the outer scurf

刮去毛　remove fuzz by scraping

净制　cleansing；cleaning

燎去毛　remove fuzz by singeing

刷去毛　remove fuzz by brushing

刷净　clean drugs by brushing away foreign matters

烫去毛　remove fuzz by scalding (usually using hot sand)

筛号　sieve number

修治　processing of Chinese crude drug

淘净　remove foreign matters from drugs by panning

挑选　sorting and choosing

筛选　selection by sifting bolting

风选　selection by winnowing (winning)

水选　select with water

剥去壳　strip the shuck

簸　fanning (winnow with a dustpan)

二、饮片切制相关术语

三分刀功，七分润功　three tenth parts is the skill of cutting and seven tenth parts is the skill of moisture (Skill of moisture is more important than that of cutting)

饮片切制　cutting of slice

切片　cut into slices

切丝　cut into slivers

切段　cut into segments (length of drug about 10—15 mm long)

切块　cut into cubes

细丝　thin slice (about 2—3mm wide)

宽丝　wide slice (about 5—10mm wide)

镑法　method for cutting drugs into very thin slices with a special knife "pangdao"

片型　piece shape of drug

极薄片　extremely thin slices (thickness Less than 0.5mm)

薄片　thin slices (thickness 1—2mm)

厚片　thick slices (thickness 2—4mm)

直片　slices cut in longitudinal section (thickness 2—4mm)

斜片　slices cut in oblique section (thickness 2—4mm)

蝴蝶片　butterfly – shaped drug slices

碾　grinding with roller

浸　soaking (in water)

浸泡　soak in (large amount of) water

浸润　moistening

浸透　soaking thoroughly

软化法　processing method of softening drugs

润软　softening by moistening

润透　moistening thoroughly

洗润　moistening after washing

闷润　softening drugs by putting the washed or moistened drugs in a sealed container

饮片　crude drugs slice processed for decoction or Chinese patent drugs

饮片干燥　drying of slices

炸心片　slices with broken center

粘连　attaching together

败片　substandard slices

翘片　warped piece

掌握水头　control the water – absorption and softening degree during softening

真空加温润药法　method for moistening crude drugs by warm – soaking under vacuum

手捏法　pinching method（for testing the degree of softening）

弯曲法　bending method（for testing the degree of softening）

穿刺法　method for examining the degree of softening by puncturing

指掐法　method for testing the degree of softness by finger pinching

阴干　drying under the shade

自然软化法　softening drugs by absorbing natural moisture

微波干燥法　method for drying drugs with microwave

水头（水性）　degree of drug softening

看水头　observing and distinguishing moisture – absorption and softening of drugs

连刀片　uncut – off herbal piece

劈开法　method for splitting drugs

热风干燥　drying with hot wind

热烘软化法　method for softening drugs by fire

热蒸软化法　method for softening drugs by steaming

伤水　excessive moisture – absorption of drugs during softening

晒干　drying under sunshine

人工干燥　artificial drying

漂　blanching and rinsing by frequently refreshing the water

漂净　removing salt，stinking smell and toxin of drugs by rinse

泡润　softening drugs by soaking them in water

喷淋法　method of spraying

喷润　moistening drugs by spraying water

加温软化法　softening crude drugs by warm – soaking

极细粉　extremely fine powder

瓜子片　melon seed – shaped drug slices

伏润法　moistening under sealed – up condition

掉边　falling off the appearance of cork

短段　length of drugs less than 9mm long

段　segment

马蹄片　horse hoof – shaped drugs slices

淋润　moistening drugs by spraying water

鳞片　scale or bud scale

柳叶片　willow leaves – shaped slices

露润　moistening drugs by absorbing natural dew

堆润　softening the crude drugs by stacking the wettish drugs with cover

三、炒法相关术语

生品　crude drugs

炒　stir – frying

炒法　method of stir – frying drugs in a pot（caldron）

炒黄　stir – frying drug to yellow

炒焦　stir – frying drug to brown

炒炭　stir – frying drug to charcoal

炒爆　make the seeds crack by stir – frying

炒断丝　stir – frying drugs till the gummy threads in the drugs are broken

炒令烟起　stir – frying the drug till the the smoke rise

炒去刺　remove the thorns of drugs by stir – frying

炒炭存性　preserve the nature of the drug after carbonization by stir – frying

炒炭止血　produce or enhance the effect of hemostasis after stir – frying drugs into charcoals in a caldron

炒香　stir – frying the drugs till they are fragrant

炒至带焦斑　stir – frying till the drug has some brown dots on the surface

炒至鼓起　stir – frying till the drugs are bulge

炒至老黄色　stir – frying till（the drugs）become dark yellow

炒至灵活　stir – frying solid adjuvants to loose

清炒（单炒）　stir – frying drugs without adjuvant

燔　broiling; setting on fire

捣碎　pounding into pieces ; stamp breaking

分档　grading

逢子必炒　the seed drugs must be stir – frying before using

麸炒　stir – frying with wheat bran

伏龙肝　clay collected from the chamber of the Chinese cook – stove

火色　coloration of heat – processed drugs

焦斑　burned dots

炮制辅料　adjuvants used for TCM processing

蛤粉 pulverized – clamshell

蛤粉炒（蛤粉烫） stir – frying with pulverized – clamshell

固体辅料 solid adjuvant

河砂 river sand

滑石粉 pulverized – talcum

滑石粉烫 stir – frying with hot pulverized – talcum

火候 optimal fire（duration and degree of heating, cooking and smelting）

火力 firing strength

加辅料炒 stir – frying with solid adjuvant

焦黑色 burned black

粳米 polished round – grained rice

糯米 polished glutinous rice

麦麸 wheat bran

米炒 stir – frying with rice

砂烫 stir – frying with hot sand

炭药 carbonized drugs

灶心土 oven earth

土炒 stir – frying with soil（stir – frying with oven earth）

陈壁土制骤补中焦 processing crude drugs with oven earth for reinforcing the function of the spleen and stomach rapidly

溏心 prepared drugs with external well done and internal half done caused by improper control of duration and degree of heating

文火 mild heating fire

中火 medium heating fire

文武火 use of mild and strong fire alternatively

武火 strong heating fire

四、炙法相关术语

米醋 rice vinegar

醋润 moistening crude drugs with rice vinegar

醋蒸 steaming crude drugs with rice vinegar

醋制 processing crude drugs with rice vinegar

醋制入肝 processing with rice vinegar for leading the drug effect into liver meridian

醋炙（醋炒） stir – frying drugs with rice vinegar

醋煮 boiling in rice vinegar

苦酒 rice vinegar

酒 wine；liquor

酒淬 quenching with liquor

酒洗　washing with rice wine

酒蒸　steaming drugs with rice wine

酒炙（酒炒）　stir – frying drugs with rice wine

白酒　liquor

米酒　rice wine

生姜汁　ginger juice

蜜麸制　stir – frying drugs with mixture of bran and honey

蜜炙　stir – frying drugs with honey

黄酒　yellow – wine；brown rice wine

乳汁炙　stir – frying drugs with milk

食盐水　water decoction of salt solution

炙法　stir – frying drugs with liquid adjuvant

炙酥　make the drug crisp by stir – frying with adjuvants

油炙　stir – frying with oil

油炸　deep – frying with oil

油脂制　stir – frying drugs with animal fats

盐水制　processing with salt solution

盐水煮　boiling in salt solution

盐炙　stir – frying drugs with salt solution

羊脂制　stir – frying with the fat of sheep

药汁制　processing with drug decoction

液体辅料　liquid adjuvant

酥油炙　stir – frying with butter

姜炙　stir – frying drugs with ginger juice or with decoction of dried ginger

米醋　rice vinegar

嫩蜜　refine honey until its temperature reaches 105℃—110 ℃

中蜜　refine honey until its temperature reaches 116℃—118℃

老蜜　refine honey until its temperature reaches 119℃—122℃

炼蜜（中蜜）　refine honey until its temperature reaches 116℃—118℃

五、煅法相关术语

明煅（敞口煅）　calcining drugs in the open air

煅淬　calcining followed by quenching

暗煅　calcining drugs in the sealed pot

醋淬　quenching by dipping in rice vinegar

醋煅淬　calcining followed by quenching with rice vinegar

直火煅　calcining drugs directly on flame

淬　quenching by dipping in water，vinegar，drug juice，etc.

焖煅　calcining drugs under sealed – up pot

煅法　calcining；calcination

煅炭存性　preserved the nature of the drug partly after calcining

制炭法　processing method for making charcoal

煅炭法　method for charcoal processing in a pot without air

煅至红透　calcine the drugs utill it become thoroughly red

扣锅煅　calcining drugs under sealed – up pot

炉口煅　calcining directly on the fire

密闭煅　calcining drugs under sealed – up condition

药汁淬　quenching with drug juice

水淬　quenching by dipping in water

六、蒸、煮、燀法相关术语

蒸法　steaming method

煮法　boiling method；cooking method

燀法　scalding method；put drugs in boiling water，then take it out，throw it into cold water rapidly，to remove the seed coat

蒸笼　steamer tub

九蒸九晒　steaming and exposing drugs to the sun alternatively for nine times

加辅料蒸法　steaming with adjuvant

姜汁蒸　steaming drugs with ginger juice

豆腐蒸　steaming with bean curd

豆腐煮（珍珠、藤黄）　cooking with bean curd

色黑如漆（熟地）　as black as lacquer

七、复制法相关术语

复制法　complex processing method

白矾制　processing with alum solution

胆汁制　processing drugs with bile

矾水煮　boiling in vitriol solution

微有麻辣感　having slight sense of numbness and pungency

内无白心　without white colored core

内无干心　without dried core found after soaking

八、发酵、发芽法相关术语

作蘖（发芽）　germination

蘖法　a method of making the seeds sprouting（budding）

作曲　processing of making leaven

发酵　fermentation

发芽率　germination rate（of seeds）

曲　leaven

发泡　foaming；foam rising

黄衣　appearance of yellow coat on the surface

九、其他制法相关术语

制霜　make crude drugs into frost – like powder

去油制霜　remove seed – oil partly by pressing to make the residue as a frost – like powder

去油制霜法 method for preparing frost – like powder by removin the oil partly

渗析制霜法　method for preparing frost – like powder through dialysis

升华制霜法　method for preparing frost – like powder through sublimation

煎煮制霜法　method for preparing frost – like powder by decocting

焙　bake over a slow fire（cook by dry heat in an oven）

鳖血炙　stir – frying drugs with turtle blood

甘草水制　processing crude drugs with decoction of Radix Glycyrrhizae

麸煨　cooking surrounded with wheat bran

干热法　dry heat processing

黑豆蒸　steaming crude drugs with black soybean juice

烘干　dry drugs in a stove or oven

烘烤　scorching on a fire

滑石粉煨　roasting drugs wrapped by hot pulverized – talcum

面煨　roasting drugs wrapped by flour paste

烘焙　drying on an oven

水飞　levigation

纸煨　roasting drugs wrapped by paper

米泔水制　processing crude drugs with rice – washed water

萝卜制　processing crude drugs with radish juice

日晒夜露　being exposed in the open air day and night

青黛拌衣　stiring and mixing with Indigo Naturalis

朱砂拌衣　stiring and mixing with cinnabar

十、中药饮片贮藏保管相关术语

风化　weathering

潮解　deliquescence

潮气　moisture in the air

虫蛀　be damaged by worms（insects）

虫蛀的　moth – eaten or worm – eaten

低温冷藏法　method for storing drugs at low temperature

发霉　mold；mildewed

发霉的　moldy

挥发　volatilizing

密闭养护法　method for maintaining the property by sealed – up

风干　air – dry

走油（泛油）　appearance of rancid oil seep onto the surface of drug

霉烂　appearance of going moldy and getting rotten

气味散失　losing of odor and flavor

摊晾　spreading and drying in the air

曝干　drying by solarizing

十一、中药炮制基本原理等相关术语

中药炮制　processing of traditional Chinese medicine（processing of traditional Chinese material media）

中药炮制学　science of processing traditional Chinese medicine（science of processing traditional Chinese material media）

制其形　change the shape of drugs by processing

制其性　weaken the over-strong character of drugs by processing

制其味　depress the flavour of drugs by processing

制其质　change the texture of drugs by processing

炒以缓其性　decrease the original property of drugs by stir – frying

胆汁制泻火　processing crude drugs with bile purging heat

贮于密闭容器　store in an airtight container

皱纹片　slice like wrinkle

走味　change of odor and flavor caused by deterioration

遵古炮制　processing abide by ancient way

胆汁制　processing crude drugs with the bile

从制　processing crude drugs with the dressing that has the same or similar property and flavour so as to promote its original property, flavour and function

四气五味　four natures and five flavors

四气　The four natures. (The four natures——cold, hot, warm and cool are summarized mainly from the body's response after Chinese medicinal herbs are taken, which are so defined in relation to the properties, cold or heat of the diseases treated)

五味　Five flavors (The five flavors of Chinese medicinal herbs refer to the five different tastes, pungent, sweet, sour, bitter and salty, which can be tasted by the tongue. With the development of the theory dealing with the medicinal properties, some flavors are summarized out of clinical actions of Chinese medicinal herbs; therefore, there is a little difference between the flavors of medicinal herbs and the tastes got by tongue)

反制　processing crude drugs with the dressing that has different or opposite property and flavor so as to decrease its original property, flavor and function

麦麸皮制抑酷性而和胃　processing crude drugs with bran manifest less property of dryness and harmonize stomach with bran

贵在适中　what really counts is properly processed

忌铁器　keeping away from iron – wares

矫臭　odour – correction

矫味　flavour – correction

解毒　detoxify

酒制升提　processing crude drugs with wine, generally manifest their effects for ascending

蜜制和中　processing crude drugs with honey for regulating and normalizing the function of stomach and spleen

蜜制益元　processing crude drugs with honey for benefit vitality

如法炮制　processing crude drugs abide by specified condition

三类分类法　three categories for TCM processing including processing with water, processing with fire, processing with both water and fire

水火共制法　processing method using both water and fire

水制法　processing method with water

生升熟降　crude drugs pertain to ascending while cooked drugs pertain to descending

生泻熟补　crude drug pertain to diarrhoea while processed drugs pertain to nourish

炮制品　processed drugs (products)

色泽　color and lustre

煨者去燥性　get rid of dry properties by roasting

味甘如饴　sweet as cerealose

吴茱萸制抑苦寒　decrease bitter and cold properties of crude drugs by processing with Fructus Evodiae juice

五类分类法　five categories for TCM processing including purification, processing with water, processing with fire, processing with both water and fire, and other processing methods

勿令犯火　avoid touching fire (avoid touching high temperature)

勿令犯水　avoid touching water

相对湿度　relative humidity

修制合度　qualified processing

修事　processing of Chinese crude drug

盐制入肾　processing crude drugs with salt manifest their effects on kidney channel

姜制发散　processing crude drugs with ginger to manifest their effects for dispersion

乳汁滋润回枯助生阴血　processing with milk for replenishing vital essence and Yin blood

相恶为制　processing crude drugs in order to damage or reduce the effects

相反为制　processing crude drugs in order to decrease the toxicity or side effects by means of auxiliary material which have different or opposite property and flavor

相杀为制　processing crude drugs in order to lessen or remove the toxicity or side effects

相须为制　processing crude drugs in order to strengthen the effects by means of auxiliary material which have similar properties or functions

相资为制　processing crude drugs in order to promote its original property, flavour and function by means of auxiliary material which have the same or similar property and flavour

参考文献
Reference

1. 丁安伟. 中药炮制学 [M]. 北京：高等教育出版社，2007.
2. 杨中林. 中药炮制学实验与指导 [M]. 北京：中国医药科技出版社，2003.
3. 国家药典委员会. 中华人民共和国药典（一部）[M]. 北京：中国医药科技出版社，2015.
4. 乔延江，王延年. 中药发酵炮制学 [M]. 北京：科学出版社，2013.
5. 王寅，李吉. 不同产地六神曲消化酶活力测定 [J]. 中药材，2003，26（7）：517 -518.
6. 石素琴. 淡豆豉炮制工艺及质量标准研究 [D]. 河北：河北医科大学，2010.